# ENDOMETRIOSIS

# ENDOMETRIOSIS

## A guide to one of the most common causes of period pain and infertility

Lyle J. Breitkopf, M.D.
and Marion Gordon Bakoulis

Thorsons
*An Imprint of* HarperCollins*Publishers*

Thorsons
An Imprint of HarperCollins*Publishers*
77–85 Fulham Palace Road
Hammersmith, London W6 8JB

First published by Thorsons 1988
Women's Health Series edition 1993
Originally published in the USA by
Prentice Hall Press, New York, 1988
1   3   5   7   9   10   8   6   4   2

A catalogue record for this book
is available from the British Library

ISBN 0 7225 2845 0

Typeset by Harper Phototypesetters Limited,
Northampton, England
Printed in Great Britain by
HarperCollinsManufacturing Glasgow

# Contents

*We dedicate this book to all women who
are coping with endometriosis, and to
their families and friends.*

# Foreword

Endometriosis is one of the commonest benign gynaecological conditions, probably occurring in two to three per cent of the overall female population and in about 10 per cent of infertile women. The condition has aroused much interest and controversy in recent years and it is now appreciated by clinicians to be much more frequent than previously thought.

Our understanding of the nature and causes of endometriosis remains one of the greatest challenges in gynaecology. There is a myriad of broad-based symptoms which the disease can produce and it may present in a variety of diverse manners throughout the reproductive years. While certain groupings of symptoms will commonly make the doctor think of endometriosis as a possible cause, more unusual symptoms and less common presentations mean that endometriosis is not initially thought of, with resultant delays in carrying out specific treatment.

While many treatments currently available have helped to relieve symptoms, this relief may not be permanent since recurrence is common in endometriosis and no 'cure' exists as yet. In recent years newer treatments, both medical and surgical, have become available which offer improved success rates for symptom relief and infertility treatment.

Our increased understanding of the disease process and the

search for a way to detect the presence of the disease at an early stage without the current need for operative (laparoscopic) diagnosis, has meant that endometriosis has been an area of intense research interest.

Despite these facts, and increased awareness of the condition among medical academics, the lay public and the general medical profession often have only a basic understanding of the nature of the disease. Although this book has been written by American authors, its content is equally applicable to the United Kingdom. This book should therefore help towards a greater understanding among sufferers of this condition with regard to its complexity and the difficulties faced by the patients and the doctors in endeavouring to detect the diagnosis and effect relief of symptoms. It should be useful in providing some insight into current areas of research and in opening up understanding of both the disease itself and the way in which endometriosis can affect the relationships of not just the patient but also those of her family and friends.

Professor R. W. Shaw, M.D., M.R.C.O.G., F.R.C.S.
*Professor of Obstetrics and Gynaecology*
*Royal Free Hospital School of Medicine,*
*London*

# Editorial preface
# by Mary Lou Ballweg

*Mary Lou Ballweg began the American Endometriosis Association, the first organization for women with endometriosis in the world, with Carolyn Keith, in 1980. She serves as its president and executive director, a staff position she took on after giving more than 2300 volunteer hours in starting the Association. Before endometriosis disabled her, she was a consultant for two large American firms and travelled extensively on business.*

When Dr Lyle J. Breitkopf asked me to write the preface to his book, I gladly agreed for three reasons. First, knowing Dr Breitkopf, I knew he would write a book that would be helpful and full of empathy for women with endometriosis, the same traits that have endeared him to hundreds of women with the disease and that led to the American Endometriosis Association's invitation to be one of our medical advisers. Second, I agreed because I view the relationship between Dr Breitkopf and the Association as a perfect example of the tremendous gains possible for all involved when a partnership occurs between a woman with endometriosis and a true professional and expert such as Dr Breitkopf. When both professionals and those with the disease work together to learn about the disease, to share what they are learning, and to make decisions with mutual respect, both the patient and the doctor come out of the process winners. The doctor need not be held responsible for the impossible – curing a disease without a cure and making decisions involving a disease for which the issues are so intensely personal that only the person *with* the disease can really make them.

And the woman, of course, is likely to make better choices when she is drawing on the information and expert advice of the doctor and on her own needs related to childbearing, sexuality, her hopes and dreams for her life, and her feelings about herself as a woman.

Third, Dr Breitkopf asked if I would address the myths surrounding endometriosis and I gladly agreed to do so as these myths have hurt women with the disease so much and also nearly had brought to a halt scientific progression and understanding of the disease over the last six decades. To understand the myths and stereotypes surrounding endometriosis, it helps to follow the trail of a typical woman with the disease. While much research remains to be done, we do know more about the 'typical' woman with endometriosis today than ever before. The Association's data registry, with more than 3000 case histories, has provided for the first time in history a solid source of information on more than 500 variables on women with endometriosis. In addition, through the work of the Association, contacts with thousands of women with the disease all across the USA add new information every day.

Let's take the story of Jennifer. Jennifer began her periods at 12. At first she didn't tell anyone about the terrible cramping, diarrhoea, nausea, and fatigue that came before and during her periods. But such symptoms were hard to hide from her mother. Her mother expressed sympathy and said that she, too, had had such problems but had been told by doctors that it would be better after she had a baby. (It wasn't, but she did not have the heart to tell Jennifer that just then.) Jenny's problems continued for several years, when her mother, unable to watch her daughter suffering any more, and hoping for some answer, took her to a fatherly, older gynaecologist. He performed Jenny's first pelvic examination and told her he could find nothing abnormal and that some girls had more difficulty adjusting to their

10

periods. He said that maybe having seen her mother in pain with her periods when she was growing up made Jenny *expect* pain.

Jenny left the doctor's office confused and feeling vaguely humiliated. Her mother felt angry at herself for subjecting her young daughter to a pelvic examination with no outcome and the implication that her daughter was not well adjusted. Both decided not to go to a doctor about the problem again. Jenny continued missing school, dates, and important family events if they happened at the time of her period. She tried every pain-killer on the market and soon found she was taking far more than the recommended amounts and still barely making it through each period. She tried to get help from the school nurse's office but she wondered if they thought she was just trying to get out of school. They would tell her to lie down and that she would probably feel better in a little while, but usually her mother had to come and get her and take her home.

By the time Jenny was 16, she was in such obvious misery that her mother took her to another doctor. This doctor said that some girls had pain but that it would go away when she had a baby. He prescribed the Pill to help alleviate the pain for now and to help get her periods on a regular schedule. Although Jenny had some bothersome side effects with the Pill, it was a tremendous blessing, for she no longer missed school, work at her part-time job, or social engagements because of her period.

By the time she was at university, after trying a number of different brands, Jenny had to go off the Pill because of side effects. For a while, she seemed okay but then the symptoms returned worse than ever. In addition, she had a new symptom she told no one about: pain with sex. She tried to live with the pain, losing her boyfriend because she couldn't explain what was happening and getting a poor grade on an exam that she had to take during her period. Drugged by the codeine that the doctor at the student health clinic prescribed for her, she managed to limp along through the bad times and then forget about them and act like a healthy college student the rest of the time. After university, at her first job, she found she couldn't work while taking the codeine and couldn't miss work as often as she had missed university lectures without losing her job. So she went back on the Pill, enduring the side effects. She met Mark, the man of her dreams, and they married.

When she was 24 they decided to try to conceive their first child. For more than two years nothing happened. At first they didn't think much about it but after a while they found they were blaming each other – Mark said they didn't have sex enough for her to get pregnant, not because she was in pain, but because her being uptight *caused* the pain. Jenny said that the amount of travelling Mark's job required made it hard to have sex at the time in her cycle when pregnancy would have been possible. They tried going on a second honeymoon as well as some home remedies suggested by well-meaning family and friends. Still no pregnancy. Finally, at 27, Jenny told her gynaecologist about the situation, even managing, finally, to briefly mention her problems with painful sex. Her gynaecologist suggested she and Mark have a few drinks before sex to help her relax. He seemed in such a hurry, and so busy, she couldn't quite bring herself to tell him they had already been doing that. Three months later, she made another appointment. This time the gynaecologist suggested she see a therapist, that she was frigid. She left the office confused and upset, and made an appointment with another gynaecologist a girlfriend had recommended. This doctor suggested infertility testing. After months of tests, she was scheduled for a laparoscopy and her problem was diagnosed: endometriosis.

Now, at the age of 29, Jenny has become a statistic in the annals of medicine. Because doctors find it hard to believe a disease could exist for years and years without their detecting it, they tend to believe the disease doesn't *start* until they diagnose it. Jenny's case, lumped together with all the other statistics, contributes to the myth that this disease occurs primarily in women in their late twenties and early thirties. All the symptoms from puberty onwards are somehow never connected with the final diagnosis.

But in reality, most women with endometriosis, like Jenny,

had typical symptoms many years before they were diagnosed. Thirty-six per cent of the women with confirmed endometriosis, whose cases are computerized in the Association's data registry, reported symptoms of the disease before the age of 20. Of these, 13 per cent experienced symptoms before the age of 15. Fifty-nine per cent reported painful symptoms before the age of 24. In studies by the Association, the British Endometriosis Society, and the Australian Victorian Endometriosis Association, in 1179 women the age of diagnosis of endometriosis was found to follow the age of first symptoms by 10 to 15 years or more. Typically, these women reported the symptoms were 'in their heads', in part because doctors have been taught by their textbooks that pain and symptoms associated with periods are mostly psychological (although these same textbooks will describe such pain and other symptoms as signs of endometriosis). The manager of an endometriosis treatment programme recently told me that about 75 per cent of women had been told their symptoms were 'in their heads', an observation corroborated by thousands of women during our eight years of work in the Association.

Jenny will also be described by some as a 'career woman' who delayed childbearing and instead chose a career. In reality, Jenny never had this choice – the disease made the choice for her. One of the basic tenets of science is that a correlation does not equal a cause; for instance, if women with endometriosis are found not to have children that does not mean that not having children causes endometriosis. Yet, amazingly, some doctors and scientists have violated this most basic principle of science in their statement that delaying childbearing could somehow cause endometriosis. Jenny, like so many other women, had symptoms of the disease long before she could attempt pregnancy.

In addition, the idea that pregnancy somehow prevents the development of endometriosis does not hold water for the women of the 1960s and 1970s with endometriosis. Millions of women, like Jenny, have spent years taking the Pill. By creating a state of pseudo-pregnancy, the pill should have resulted in far less endometriosis today if, indeed, pregnancy is a preventative for endometriosis.

Although it has now been thoroughly discredited, another myth about endometriosis surfaces enough to be addressed – the idea that pregnancy *cures* the disease. From the beginnings of the Association, women with endometriosis who had been pregnant and still had the disease were part of our group. Dr Donald Chatman disproved this myth and a couple of others in an important study in which he documented endometriosis in teenagers who had had babies before the age of 17!

This myth probably developed because the worst symptoms of endometriosis – the pain that occurs with the monthly period – cannot occur when one is pregnant and not having periods. However, to leap from that observation to the statement that pregnancy *cures* the disease is a leap of faith with no scientific evidence to back it up. In fact, what little scientific evidence on pregnancy and endometriosis there is leads more in the other direction – that the disease process continues in pregnancy. The first statements on pregnancy and endometriosis date back to 1922, but the first rigid study of what actually happens to endometrial implants during pregnancy was not done until 1967. The 1967 study found that in some cases symptoms increased during pregnancy; in others they decreased. In 12 of the 25 cases studied, the implants grew larger during pregnancy; in an additional six cases they grew larger in the post partum period. Some of the endometriomas (cysts) grew and then receded during the pregnancies; others diminished in size initially and then began to grow again. The authors of the study concluded that the behaviour of endometriosis during pregnancy was extremely variable and that 'patients alleged to exhibit permanent regression following pregnancy are encountered much less frequently than patients with manifestly persistent disease'.

In an important preliminary study conducted by Carolyn Ansell and Catherine Gorchoff of the Yale School of Nursing Midwifery with the assistance of the American Endometriosis Association and reported in the Association's newsletter, the actual pregnancy experiences of women with endometriosis were studied. The results on 187 pregnancies were astounding:

the women experienced *multiple* discomforts during their pregnancies, a high incidence of dysfunctional labour, an extremely high rate of post-partum depression, return of symptoms with the return of periods, and a faster return of symptoms in those who did not breast-feed. The study also backed-up findings of high rates of miscarriage and ectopic pregnancy in women with endometriosis.

Finally, it seems the ethical issues are often overlooked in this particular myth about endometriosis. How profoundly disrespectful of life – the woman's and the potential child's – to suggest to someone that they have a baby to 'cure' a disease! To suggest to women, whether they be in their teens or older; single or coupled; heterosexual, gay, or celibate; in a relationship capable of sustaining a child or not; or even whether they *want* a child or not, that they have a child because they have a disease seems ludicrous even if it *did* cure the disease. That this 'treatment' is 'prescribed' so often, as is reported by thousands of women to the Association, is scandalous. Moreover, several important studies, including one of the Association's, have found that in the most severe cases of endometriosis, the risk of other family members having the disease (*and* other health problems, as documented by additional studies) is increased. This awareness is not yet widespread but it will present a devastating moral dilemma if doctors and others perpetuate the pregnancy-cure myth. That dilemma, to 'cure' one's own disease by taking the risk of passing it and other problems on to a child is too horrible to think about.

There are many other myths about endometriosis, but I'll examine only two more here as they show so clearly how the myths evolved without scientific validation. First, there is the myth that says women with endometriosis are underweight mesomorphs – trim, slender women. 'How I wish that were true', a member recently commented to me. A very simple study comparing the weights and heights of women with endometriosis, data that appear in every medical chart, could have shown whether women with endometriosis do indeed tend toward slenderness. And when one reads quotes from experts about the body type of women with endometriosis, one automatically assumes this has been done. But, in fact, it was not done until seven infertility clinics carried out such a study and reported it in 1986. It found women with endometriosis do *not* differ in weight from women without endometriosis (but they do tend to be slightly taller).

One has to wonder why endometriosis seems to have been the free-for-all women's disease, the area in which science stops and speculation runs rampant. I believe it is because in endometriosis one can find a microcosm of society's attitudes about women. The disease is intricately wrapped up in the most intensely female experiences and the most taboo-laden areas about women. Endometriosis involves the defining experiences of being female: menstruation, female sexuality, childbearing. Being a child of the 1960s when we invented slogans such as 'Make love, nor war', wore see-through blouses and no bras, and the Pill made 'free love' more possible for women than before, I was not prepared for the shock of discovering, as I began my work to help myself and other women with endometriosis, how taboo the subjects of menstruation and female sexuality still were. I found I couldn't go into corporate or foundation boardrooms and explain endometriosis and expect to get a grant for our work. The sudden silence when the word 'menstruation' was used told me very clearly what the problem was.

And recently, working on a special issue of the Association's newsletter on endometriosis and male partners and coping with painful sex, I again realized how taboo and little known the realities of female sexuality are. The letters of women describing the attitudes of the men in their lives related to painful intercourse, one of the most common symptoms of endometriosis, showed ignorance and power struggles that would be problems even without endometriosis. But because of the disease, women with endometriosis cannot escape these problems. Add to this all the other issues of the disease and it's small wonder many women with endometriosis find their marriages dissolve.

The letters describe how many of the men find it hard to

believe that endometriosis can cause severe pain with intercourse, then go on to show that the men (and the women, too, sometimes) do not understand *normal* female sexuality, much less the complications of endometriosis. For instance, many people believe that the vagina is an open space always ready for a man the woman loves and many anatomic drawings incorrectly depict the vagina this way. In reality the walls of the vagina normally touch each other until foreplay and arousal balloon them out. Abrupt penetration causes discomfort even for a woman without endometriosis if she is not ready for intercourse. For a woman with endometriosis, it can cause excruciating pain. Another belief of many people that contributes to sexual problems for all women but makes life miserable for women with endometriosis is the widespread lack of awareness that lubrication is the female equivalent of erection. When these basics of female sexuality are not understood, as is so clear from many of the letters, the adjustment necessary to eliminate pain due to endometrial implants on the ligaments of the uterus or in the cul-de-sac are beyond the capability of the couple.

To make matters even worse, the letters often show how many men *define* sex as intercourse instead of a whole range of intimate behaviours between partners. This equation of sex and intercourse and, in some cases, unwillingness by men to adapt to the needs of a woman with endometriosis to make it possible for her to be sexual without pain (such as the woman on top so she can control the depth of penetration, or other sexual activities besides intercourse), was another shock to me. I had naively thought the 'sexual revolution' of the 1960s had changed all that. It didn't. But even that isn't the whole picture of what many women with endometriosis have to deal with in this most intimate aspect of their lives. Add to this terribly difficult situation the doctors who are, unfortunately, offered little or no training on painful sex in medical school yet are willing to tell a woman and her husband that the woman is frigid instead of properly diagnosing her endometriosis, and you have a clear case of males defining the female realities of female sexuality and endometriosis.

The power to define reality is really the power that is at the heart of the myth-making about endometriosis. Until women with the disease banded together and started working with each other and very special and wise doctors such as Dr Breitkopf, that power combined with taboos about women and cultural biases to create a 'reality' about endometriosis that was myth and to bring new scientific understanding to a halt. A final example is the myth that endometriosis is a white woman's disease. Why? Because, as a leading gynaecologist involved internationally in training other gynaecologists confided to me at the beginning of the Association, gynaecologists would almost automatically diagnose a black woman with symptoms of endometriosis as having pelvic inflammatory disease (PID). The underlying reason was an assumption that black women were sexually promiscuous (which is a known factor in contracting gonorrhoea and PID). These women then were accounted for, statistically, in the numbers of women with PID, not endometriosis, further perpetuating the myth that black women did not get endometriosis but PID! Except, the numbers, now in the guise of science, could not be accused of racism! And those numbers, based on racism, reinforced the scientific 'truth' that black women did not get endometriosis.

It's no wonder, with so much myth, taboo, and confusion surrounding endometriosis, that no major breakthroughs in understanding the disease, no new theories about its development, or new conceptual frameworks for treatment evolved from the 1920s to the 1980s. And so I make an appeal that may seem strange coming from a lay person, and that is an appeal to return to science, *true* science, on endometriosis. Let's look at the disease with new eyes, throw out the socio-economic myths and taboos and assumptions about women, and start over. Women with endometriosis stand ready to be partners in the progress inevitable from this fresh start.

# Introduction

This book has been many years in the making. It was quite a while, however, before pen was actually put to paper.

I have been treating endometriosis for 25 years, since the days when the condition was known to only a few doctors and their unfortunate patients as the 'career woman's disease' and treated – even when it was properly diagnosed – with aspirin, birth control pills and major surgery. The first major impetus to write a book about endometriosis came in the form of a patient. Bertine Columbo was in her early 30s when I met her in 1981, at the time that I first diagnosed her case of endometriosis. Her story was distressingly familiar: she had been in pain for years and she and her husband were unable to conceive a child. She told me that she had visited 17 doctors in an attempt to diagnose and treat her condition.

Bertine's case was different from that of most other patients, however, in one important respect. Once she was diagnosed with endometriosis, she became extremely open about her condition. She told her family and friends exactly what was wrong with her. Most people had never head of endometriosis and didn't know what to make of the strange-sounding disorder. But they sympathized with Bertine, and she in turn understood the situation of other women who she later learned had the same condition.

Eventually Bertine founded the New York City branch of the Endometriosis Association, a nationwide group of patients, their families, and friends founded to provide support, information, and referrals concerning endometriosis. Because of my activities in the association (I served as consultant to the group in 1982), we remained in touch. She would often tell me that she longed to share with a wide audience the story of her long struggle to arrive at a diagnosis for her condition. She felt that there were so many misconceptions about endometriosis and so many women who suffered from the condition without even knowing it.

Several times she suggested that I write a book about my experience diagnosing and treating hundreds of patients and fill the large gaps in the public's knowledge about who suffers from endometriosis, how the condition affects women and their families, and what can be done about it. She stressed the immediate importance of educating the public, reminding me that I had hundreds of case histories which I could use as examples of how the disease affects women and how they deal with it.

I knew Bertine was right. I had seen first-hand, over and over, how endometriosis affected the day-to-day lives of hundreds of women, and I knew that millions of other patients and their families were having the same sort of experiences. Ten million women in the USA, and two million in Britain, have endometriosis at any given time, and most of them will never realize it until they are diagnosed with the condition, and even then they receive very little information and support. In short, I knew that the need was there, but somehow I could never find the time to devote to putting such information together into a book.

Finally, in the autumn of 1985, it seemed that the project could not wait any longer. A magazine interviewed me and ran an article on endometriosis. It stressed the mysterious nature of the disease, the fact that it had no cure other than menopause, and that many cases went unrecognized for years because of the difficulty of diagnosis.

The week after the article appeared hundreds of letters began to pour into my office. Some were writing to express relief that the symptoms they'd suffered for so long actually had a name; some wrote to feel solidarity with other sufferers; some were thanking me for providing information for a suffering family member or friend. Almost all, however, were hungry for information about their condition. It was a powerful reminder of what I already knew to be true, that women with endometriosis needed information.

I also knew that the medical technology affecting diagnosis and treatment of the condition was rapidly changing. Doctors were now able to recognize and classify endometriosis at earlier stages and offer patients faster and less debilitating treatments. I knew of the potential for even better tests, and even the possibility of a preventive vaccine for the condition.

The changes were exciting and showed even more promise for the future. I wanted endometriosis patients and their families and friends to learn that there was good news.

So finally, I teamed up with Marion Gordon Bakoulis, a magazine writer and editor with a special interest in women's reproductive health. We agreed to shape the book around the stories of actual patients, women either I or a close colleague had treated, whose cases had met with varying degrees of success.

These women's stories are the essence of this book. We have brought them together to provide a real life picture of the disease, to show you not just what happens inside the body of a woman with endometriosis but how these changes affect her on the outside – her marriage, job, relationships, and plans to have children.

You will see that we don't look at the situation through rose-coloured glasses. On the other hand, we don't feel it is enough just to paint pictures of pain and suffering. We have tried to offer a realistic picture of life with endometriosis, which, as you may well know, can be a tough experience, full of pain, and the possibility – or, in many cases, the reality – of infertility. But the real picture is also filled with hope – hope of new treatments and earlier detection, and of more support and understanding of the condition from family, friends, and all of society. Rather than dwelling on the painful aspects of the condition that you probably already know very well, we focus on offering solutions.

We hope you will read and use this book as a guide for living with endometriosis, whether you have it yourself, think that you may, or know someone who has it. We think you will find it helpful in accepting and controlling your condition.

# Acknowledgements

Lyle J. Breitkopf, MD would like to thank Bertine Columbo, a longtime patient whose idea this book first was and whose persistent encouragement helped it become a reality; and Maria Perper, former president of the Greater New York branch of the Endometriosis Association and unfailing source of enthusiasm and encouragement. Thank you both for all your support.

Marion Gordon Bakoulis wants to thank her family and friends for their patience through all those weekends when the hours on the word processor had to come first, and for their sincere interest in and enthusiasm for this project. A special thanks to Rona Cherry for planting the seed that set this project in motion.

From both of us, our abundant gratitude to our literary agent, Meredith Bernstein, who supported our work through its completion and offered practical, straightforward advice at several stages; and to P. J. Dempsey, our editor, whose skill in bringing our efforts to fruition has been matched only by her infinite patience and understanding at every step.

# Prologue

# ONE PATIENT'S STORY

At first, Jeanne's pain came and went, and it didn't concern her all that much. She'd feel a twinge now and then when she rolled over on her side after having intercourse with her husband, Ned. Or her lower back might ache a bit the day she started her period – but what woman didn't have occasional menstrual cramps? And since she never had cramps in her teens like so many of her friends, Jeanne, who was now almost 31 considered herself lucky and figured it was now her turn to deal with monthly period cramps.

Although she hardly noticed the pain, Jeanne did mention it to her gynaecologist after her yearly examination. He had performed the standard manual pelvic examination and told her he had not detected any problem. She shouldn't worry.

Feeling reassured, Jeanne went on with her life, working as an assistant vice-president at a bank, pursuing her hobbies of sailing, studying modern dance, and oil painting. She'd just been promoted at work, after months of putting in long hours on extra assignments. The effort had put her under some stress, but now she felt only joy that it had all paid off.

But one winter night, Jeanne could no longer ignore her pain, which had been becoming increasingly worse. In particular, she found that the pain in her lower back and abdomen during intercourse had become almost unbearable, especially around the time of her period.

One night when Ned penetrated her, Jeanne yelled out in pain. She pushed him away and drew her knees to her chest against the pain in her lower abdomen and across the small of her back. She felt such a terrible pain, as if something was bound up and trying to tear loose.

Ned wanted to call a doctor. Jeanne insisted she was fine and made sure there was no blood. She promised to call her gynaecologist first thing in the morning.

She didn't tell him that she'd been feeling pain for months whenever they made love, a dull but persistent ache that dwindled away afterwards each time.

Jeanne made an appointment the next morning to see her doctor, who was unable to schedule her until a week later. By then she had finished her period, and her pain had disappeared.

During the examination the doctor probed her abdomen, inserted a speculum into her vagina to view her cervix. He completed the examination by gently pressing her uterus and ovaries. Jeanne reported that she felt no pain.

The doctor told her that nothing was wrong. His guess was that it was just menstrual cramps. He suggested that she take aspirin and use a hot compress on her back.

Jeanne reported the news to Ned, who shrugged and said that he hoped it wouldn't happen again.

But as Jeanne's period approached the next month her pain returned. She and Ned decided not to have intercourse for a few nights since they were both worried that Jeanne would experience the same excruciating pain as before. The next month she was out of town on a business trip around the time of her period. Even without sex, though, the pain seemed to be worse.

By the next month both Jeanne and Ned were frustrated and worried. But she reminded him that her doctor had said that nothing was wrong. Jeanne didn't like to take aspirin too often, so she and Ned continued to refrain from intercourse around the time of her period. Neither of them was very enthusiastic about this plan, but they tolerated it for a few months.

Jeanne, however, could not ignore the fact that her pain was getting worse. And another worry nagged at her: after nearly a year of regular, unprotected intercourse, she was not pregnant. If anything, her period seemed to be getting heavier each month. She made another appointment with her gynaecologist. He examined her again and gave her a prescription for a stronger painkiller than the aspirin.

The doctor dismissed her worries about possible infertility. 'Everyone wants to have a baby these days,' he said. 'Wait another six months, at least.'

Jeanne knew for certain that her pain was worse. She now dreaded having intercourse with Ned for a full two weeks before her period. And the pain didn't merely come during sex, it was just at its worst then. Sometimes, though, Jeanne would have to leave her desk at work and spend 15 minutes in the bathroom, sitting on the toilet and leaning forward to ease the ache across the small of her back.

The pain exhausted her. It kept her awake late into the night, and she'd be so tired at work the next afternoon that she would leave work at 5 p.m. with the secretaries, instead of staying late with the other executives to put in her time on important assignments. She would come home, pour herself a glass of wine, take a painkiller, lie down on the couch, and wait for Ned to come home.

'What's a bank executive doing home at this hour?' he would say, trying to get her to laugh. She would barely smile. She took painkillers every day, but they no longer seemed to help. Sometimes she would drink four glasses of wine in an evening so she could finally fall asleep.

Once she postponed an important business trip because it fell around the time of her period. She was afraid the pain would incapacitate her. When she returned home Ned was waiting for her in the living room. He quietly told her that their marriage 'couldn't go on like this'. They hadn't made love in almost a month, and Jeanne was constantly irritated, tired, and complaining about the pain. Ned began accusing her of using her complaints to cover up the fact that she was having an affair, which wasn't true. They decided to see a marriage counsellor.

The therapist they went to see listened to Ned and Jeanne's story, then gave Jeanne a card with the name of yet another gynaecologist. The next morning Jeanne called and scheduled an appointment.

It was a few days before she was due to get her period. The doctor's light touch on her abdomen made her cry out in pain.

This doctor suggested she start taking birth control pills. This made no sense to Jeanne since her prime objective was to get pregnant. The only explanation offered was, 'You have to get well first.'

Jeanne had been on the Pill for a while at university. She had gained weight and become so depressed that she switched back to the diaphragm after six months. This time was just as bad. First her weight ballooned – she gained five, ten, 20 pounds. Then came bouts of depression that caused her to burst into tears at the slightest provocation – a lost memo on her desk, a ladder in her tights. She called her doctor and told him that she couldn't stay on the medication anymore but that the pain hadn't been as bad these past few months. Her doctor urged her to keep taking the Pill for a few more months.

One night a few weeks later Ned and Jeanne were getting ready for bed. They had barely touched each other in months, but that night as Ned leaned over to kiss her goodnight, Jeanne caught him in a passionate embrace. They made love for hours. Jeanne felt no pain, though her period was only a week away.

A few days later, after they had again had intercourse, Ned brought up the subject of starting a family. By this time Jeanne was almost 34, and she and Ned had always planned to have at least two children.

So without telling her doctor, Jeanne stopped taking the birth control pills. She dropped back to her normal weight. For a few weeks the pain remained at bay. Within two months, however, it was back.

Again, Jeanne found intercourse impossible. Again she grew haggard, coming home from work early and staying awake late when the pain was at its worst. She continued to try and control her pain by drinking and taking painkillers, and was so distracted that she didn't notice that Ned often came home late. One night however, he confessed that he was having an affair. Instead of getting angry, Jeanne cried and begged him not to leave her. She felt as though her life was falling to pieces.

It got worse and worse. Jeanne was convinced she was going to lose both her marriage and her job. She didn't want to talk to a close friend, but finally she confided everything to a friend from work.

This woman gave her the name of yet another gynaecologist. She said that she had heard great things about him from another friend who went to him the year before, when she had endometriosis.

'What?' asked Jeanne.

The first thing this doctor did was hand Jeanne a pamphlet. Jeanne shook her head, baffled, as she read the description of the condition. 'Endometriosis is the implantation of tissue resembling the endometrium, or lining of the uterus, on other parts of the body outside that organ.'

It sounded bizarre to Jeanne. She wondered how in the world such a thing would happen to an otherwise perfectly healthy 33-year-old woman. Then she started to read about the condition's symptoms: 'Endometriosis is characterized by pelvic pain around the time of menstruation, painful intercourse, and excessive menstrual flow. Infertility results in 50 per cent of all cases.'

The doctor tried to perform a manual pelvic examination, but Jeanne felt so much pain that he soon asked her to get dressed and come into his office.

Jeanne was grilled with questions. The doctor wanted to know when the pain had first occurred. When and where did she feel it? Were her bowel movements painful? Did she have painful, irregular, or excessive menstrual periods? Did she ever feel pain at mid-cycle? Did she get backaches? How about constipation? Spotting between periods?

Jeanne answered all the doctor's questions. Rather than feel annoyed or threatened, she actually experienced an immense sense of excitement and hope over the fact that someone finally seemed to be trying to unravel the mystery of her terrible ailment. She mentioned as well that she had been trying to get pregnant for over two years.

The doctor took copious notes on everything Jeanne said. Then he sighed, looked at the paper, at her, and began to explain.

Many things could be causing her symptoms. The only way to find out for sure what is wrong is to perform a laparoscopy. He described an operation in which Jeanne would be under anaesthesic and the doctor would make a small incision just below the navel to insert a fibre-optic tube to view the abdominal cavity and reproductive organs.

'It's a simple procedure, and I strongly recommend it,' he said, 'but it is surgery. What you may want to do is wait and keep a diary of your symptoms for several months.'

But all Jeanne wanted to do at this point was to find out what was wrong with her and have it treated.

Her surgery was scheduled for the following week, first thing in the morning. As she was recovering from the operation, her doctor told her that she had extensive endometriosis with adhesions covering the fallopian tubes and ovaries, the utero-sacral ligaments, and bowel. This was the cause of the pain and infertility. He had cauterized several large cysts, but recommended she start a course of the drug danocrine.

Jeanne was so drowsy that the words barely made sense. One fact registered, however: her disease was real. It had a name. The next day, when she was more alert, she and Ned went back for a consultation. The doctor told them that Jeanne's case was quite advanced ('stage three' he informed them); however, he had seen others like it in which the woman had gone on to conceive and bear children.

Jeanne was given a prescription for a medication called Danazol, which would shrink the remaining endometrial implants. She was warned of possible side effects: weight gain, deepening of the voice, growth of facial hair, and acne.

Jeanne took Danazol twice a day for six months. Her pain

disappeared completely. She also suffered all the side effects her doctor had mentioned, as well as depression, occasional headaches, and fatigue. She knew she was hard to live with. She did not become pregnant, but she and Ned were having intercourse so seldom that she wasn't surprised. One day Ned told her that he couldn't deal with her problems anymore and thought it best if he moved out for a while. Jeanne felt too sick and tired to argue.

When she finally stopped taking Danazol, she felt no pain for a few months. She felt good about herself. She got a raise at work, and Ned moved back in. For the first time in years she started to feel hopeful about herself and her future.

One month she missed her period. A pregnancy test confirmed that she was at last expecting a child. Two months later, however, Jeanne had a miscarriage.

She felt more discouraged than ever. It hardly helped that her doctor told her that several studies showed that endometriosis increased the rate of miscarriage, but that the fact that she was able to get pregnant was an encouraging sign. However, ultrasound revealed that endometrial growths still bound Jeanne's uterus, fallopian tubes, ovaries, and lower bowel. She urged the doctor to do another operation, but he did not want to risk damaging the organs. He suggested that she undergo another course of Danazol, but she thought about the side effects and said no to that.

The doctor urged Jeanne to get in touch with the local branch of the Endometriosis Association. Jeanne did, and started to receive the group's monthly newsletter. For the first time, she learned that as many as two million British women suffered from the condition. She couldn't believe it – *two million women*. She wondered what was being done to find better treatments for endometriosis and why, for that matter, it had taken doctors years to even diagnose her case.

She joined a support group and spent her free time at the library reading whatever literature she could find on the condition – which wasn't very much.

Jeanne's pain quickly became unbearable once again, and on

the advice of the women in her support group, she decided to take Danazol for another six months. From what she could gather, it was the best available treatment.

One woman referred her to a doctor who advocated the use of a new type of laser surgery that 'vaporized' endometrial growths, and Jeanne sent him a letter asking for help. By this time Ned and Jeanne had separated again.

In her letter to the doctor Jeanne wrote, 'I can accept the fact that I probably will never have children. I know that any further treatment may be difficult and expensive and have side effects. I can take that, but I just can't take any more pain.'

Jeanne is fictional, a composite of many endometriosis patients I have treated and heard about over the years. Her condition, though, is very real. Not only that, but endometriosis is thought to affect up to 30 per cent of all menstruating women.

What exactly is this condition? Who gets it? How is it treated?

These questions, and many others, will be explored in this book.

# Chapter 1

# AN OVERVIEW

I know that I'm just one of many women who have this disease.

*A 34-year-old patient*

In beginning any discussion on endometriosis, it is easiest to mention first those few things we know for certain about the condition. It is defined as the presence of tissue resembling the

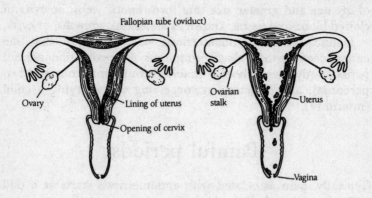

*Figure 1(a)* Thickening of endometrial lining; (*b*) Endometrial lining being shed normally.

endometrium, or lining of the uterus, outside that organ. You might want to think of it as a normal part of the body located in an abnormal place.

Inside the uterus, the endometrium thickens each month after menstruation as the uterus prepares again to receive a fertilized egg. If the egg is not fertilized, of course, the endometrial lining is not needed, so it leaves the body through the vagina as menstrual flow. This process, as we know, is repeated over and over, with a new lining growing and being shed each month, except during pregnancy, from puberty to menopause.

It is not clear how tissue resembling the endometrium grows outside that organ – nor even if endometrial growths have anything to do with the endometrium, though the theory that they are somehow related is widely accepted. (You'll find a complete discussion of the theories of what causes the condition in Chapter 3.)

Some endometrial implants seem to respond to the same hormonal changes that signal to the endometrium what to do each month. Like the lining, the implants seem to, in most cases, thicken, grow, and bleed each month. Unlike the endometrium, however, the endometrial tissue cannot leave the body through menstruation. Instead, the monthly bleeding produces implants of greater and greater size that form knots, webs, or cysts of clotted blood and tissue, known as adhesions, growths, or cysts.

Jeanne's case of endometriosis was typical in that she experienced the three classic symptoms of the condition: painful periods (dysmenorrhoea), pain during intercourse (dyspareunia), and difficulty in conceiving and carrying a child (infertility).

# Painful periods

Typically, pain associated with endometriosis starts as a dull ache for several days each month around the time of menstruation. As the condition progresses, however, a woman may feel pain throughout the month, and, for some patients, the pain appears to be unrelated to menstruation even from the beginning.

# Pain during intercourse

Pain during intercourse again may start as mild and occasional and later become excruciating. This is because the uterus becomes so rigidly held by adhesions to the abdominal cavity wall that any movement is painful. Surgery may temporarily improve the condition but tends to leave scars that eventually result in the growth of more adhesions, and the development of more pain.

Endometriosis patients who develop adhesions around the bowel and bladder may have painful bowel movements and be more prone to urinary tract infections. Rectal bleeding and constipation may be signs that the adhesions have grown so large around the colon that they threaten to shut off the bowel. Again, surgery can correct the condition but usually only temporarily.

# Infertility

Infertility results from endometriosis when adhesions block the fallopian tubes or ovaries. When this happens, either an egg is not released or it is blocked from travelling down the tube to the uterus. For this reason, endometriosis increases a woman's chance of having an ectopic pregnacy, which happens when a fertilized egg attaches itself outside the uterus. The condition is potentially fatal.

Many women remain infertile even after treatment for endometriosis because cysts on the ovaries have permanently destroyed their ability to produce and release an egg. Infertility may even occur in the absence of adhesions in this area; many doctors believe that this is due to changes in hormone levels that the condition seems to cause. Fertility specialists estimate that endometriosis accounts for 20 to 40 per cent of all cases of infertility, affecting millions of couples. In many cases, the infertility that results from endometriosis causes more anguish for patients than the condition itself. (See Chapter 9 for a complete discussion of infertility associated with endometriosis.)

Even without infertility, it is clear that endometriosis represents a serious health problem for women of reproductive age. This has ramifications for all of society. Women lose millions of work days each year due to absenteeism because of the condition.

Since the cause of endometriosis is not known (although theories abound), and the only permanent cure is hysterectomy, the disease is mysterious and frustrating to patients and their families. If you have, or someone you know well has, endometriosis you already know something of the frustration. It's not unusual for endometriosis to cause stress in relationships and even to be a factor in the break up of marriages. The stresses in Jeanne's life that resulted from her condition are experienced by millions of women.

The surprising thing is that most women – even those with a university education – have never even heard of endometriosis. And even those who have – if they know someone with the condition, have it themselves, or have read an article or two about it in a women's magazine or the general press – often have mistaken notions about it. Some believe it's very rare, or deadly, or both.

Endometriosis is neither. The chances are that someone you know has endometriosis. You may even have it yourself and not know it. If you do, you certainly won't die from it, or even become terribly ill, but it *will* affect the quality of your life. You'll probably feel pain at some point, and you may have trouble having a child.

In October 1985, a magazine published an interview with me about my work in diagnosing and treating endometriosis. I was warned by the editors that the article would generate a flood of mail – even though my address was not printed in the magazine – but I was unprepared for the deluge that poured into my office. I read and have saved all of those letters. They tell the stories of women all over the world who have suffered with endometriosis. Excerpts from many of the letters are printed here for the first time, with names and identifying details omitted to protect the individuals' privacy. Many of the women (and in some cases their husbands or boyfriends) wrote asking questions about the condition, treatment options, doctors, clinics, and support groups in their area. Others wrote simply to share their stories – from the all-too-familiar to the highly unusual – such as the woman who vomited blood after intercourse for years until it was finally determined that she had extensive endometriosis in her lung. You will find the stories of dozens of the women who took the trouble to write in response to my original article interspersed throughout this book.

If you have endometriosis, you probably have a number of questions about it. As you may have already discovered, your doctor does not have all the answers. We hope that this book will provide many of the answers you need and raise questions that you may not have thought of. With endometriosis, there are still many questions to which we don't have answers. We can't tell you why you, and not your friend or co-worker, has the condition. We don't know for sure whether you will be better in three months and whether you will be able to get pregnant next year.

What this book does do is share with you the stories of dozens of women who have, or have had, endometriosis. We've changed the women's names and in some cases a few details to protect their privacy, but all the stories are based on actual medical histories of patients I've either treated or learned of through other doctors.

We tell you how the patients' condition affected them, how it was diagnosed and treated, and what happened as a result. In many cases, as we do in the story of Jeanne, we leave the woman's case history unfinished. We do this because this is the way treatment often ends for women with endometriosis. They have surgery and drug treatment, experience relief, but then their symptoms recur. They are left having to choose between further treatment – sometimes even complete hysterectomy –

or learning simply to live with their condition. This book will not attempt to tell these women – or tell you – what to do but will provide examples you may want to follow.

It can be a tremendous help to know that you are not alone with endometriosis. One woman who responded to the magazine article said simply: 'I don't feel so alone and depressed. I'm not the only one who has this monster.'

This book will also tell you what studies have found out about how the condition may be caused and, more importantly, which avenues of medical research and clinical practice are showing the most promise for finding better treatments and cures. Endometriosis is becoming an important area of medical research and practice, and we report on the state-of-the-art research and treatment.

Although the endometriosis picture sometimes looks bleak, there has been much progress in dealing with the problem. We've learned so much about the condition, just in the past few years. We know that it occurs in women of all ages, races and socio-economic backgrounds, not just, as many experts used to believe, in white, well-off 'career' women who have put off having children (although delayed childbearing can make the condition worse in a woman who already has it).

If you have endometriosis, we know that you do not want false promises about your condition. Many of your questions may have disturbing answers that contradict the cheery reassurances you have heard from friends, doctors, and even published articles. For example, many women are told that pregnancy 'cures' endometriosis. The fact is that while pregnancy halts the growth of endometrial implants, studies have shown that the condition recurs after pregnancy in at least 50 per cent of all cases.

Although the cause of endometriosis is a mystery, there is quite a bit of evidence that a woman whose mother, grandmother, sister, or daughter had or has it is up to eight times as likely as the average woman to develop the condition herself.

The questions are many, and while the answers often are sketchy, we have been learning a great deal about endometriosis.

We think women need more answers – not only women who have endometriosis, but anyone who knows someone who has it, or any woman who simply cares about her body and good health.

We think you'll find many more of the answers to your questions about endometriosis in the following chapters, beginning with the importance of having a good relationship with your doctor.

# Chapter 2

# THE ENDOMETRIOSIS PATIENT AND HER DOCTOR

> He didn't say much, as doctors usually do, and said that I
> needed to have ultrasound right away. I decided to speak up and
> I asked him. 'Exactly what are your feelings about the exam-
> ination?' His reply: 'It looks like endometriosis again.' I was
> crushed, and on the 40 minute drive home, I just broke down.
>
> *A 22-year-old patient*

Some time ago, one doctor I know performed the following
study: he videotaped several conversations with patients during
which he explained the reasons for an upcoming surgical
procedure, how it would be carried out, what the risks were, and
what the post-operative course would be. The patients were
allowed to ask questions and discuss their operation as
extensively as they wished.

Following the surgery the patients viewed the tapes, and then
the doctor interviewed them to get their reactions. He was
surprised to find that many of the patients did not remember
much of their pre-operative conversation. In fact, many of them
did not even remember that the meeting had taken place. They
were shocked when they saw the tapes re-played and heard their
own voices talking about their upcoming surgery.

This is a classic example of poor communication between patient and doctor. If you have endometriosis, it is more crucial than in many other diseases for you and your doctor to communicate effectively with one another.

But what is meant by effective communication, why is it so important, and what can patients and their physicians do to make sure it is maintained?

Everyone has an idea of what the doctor-patient relationship is like. In many cases this idea is quite different from what they feel the relationship *should* be like. Endometriosis is a condition that forces you into a more intense relationship with your doctor than you may have ever had before. You may be in weekly, and sometimes even daily, contact with each other for weeks, months, or years and become partners in decisions affecting your family, career, and sex life. So it stands to reason that you would want to work to establish and maintain a good relationship with this doctor.

Now that you know how important a good relationship with your doctor is, how do you go about achieving it? First of all, in a good doctor-patient relationship there is open communication and trust on both sides. In order for you and your doctor to communicate well – that means each of you being able both to talk freely *and* listen – you have to feel certain positive things about one another.

I feel that your relationship with your doctor is positive and productive when:

- You can trust his or her level of knowledge
- You are confident in his or her technical skills
- You feel comfortable enough to ask all the questions you have, knowing that the doctor will not be annoyed or threatened by them or by you
- You feel that your doctor does not resent taking the time to explain things to you carefully and will listen closely as you describe all your symptoms and concerns.

In other words, you should expect your doctor to be not only competent in treating your condition but caring and compassionate as well. Most endometriosis patients feel these traits are especially important in treating a condition that affects very personal and emotional aspects of their lives – sexuality, family planning, and fertility – and may last for years.

Here are some comments from patients with endometriosis who feel they have a good relationship with their doctor:

> Beyond his medical expertise, he is a sensitive and supportive person. He is well-informed and willing to share updated medical research on issues relevant to today's woman. He is most patient and understanding in discussing the emotional impact of medical issues.

> He values a well-informed patient, welcomes questions, and realizes that the responsibility for choices concerning my medical options remains *mine*, not his. During my pre-surgery visit, when he had finished answering my long list of questions to my satisfaction, I said, 'What more could I ask for?' His reply: 'What *less* could you be satisfied with?'

> She listens to my concerns and displays genuine concern and compassion. In addition, she clearly provides a lot of objective information about my condition, answers questions, and proceeds in her treatment in a logical, cautious manner. She believes patients should be involved in their health care.

In establishing a good relationship with a doctor during your treatment of endometriosis, it's important to keep in mind not only your needs and wishes but your doctor's as well. I've found that many, if not most, patients have a hard time doing this. Most doctors feel that a good doctor-patient relationship is one in which:

- The patient is honest about her symptoms and other aspects of her life that may touch on her condition
- The patient takes the time to learn about her body and the specific disease process

- The patient presents any relevant information in an organized and coherent way. Does she plan to have children, for example, or does she know of other cases of endometriosis in her family?
- The patient is open about her needs, fears, and concerns as they affect her condition and treatment. For example, is she afraid of a hospital stay, reluctant to take a certain type of medication, or worried about an operation? A doctor needs to know these things
- The patient follows the treatment plan she and the doctor agree upon and discusses the possibility of any changes
- The patient does not have unrealistic expectations of what a doctor can do. This is especially important with endometriosis, which is a chronic condition that may respond unexpectedly or incompletely to even the best available treatment.

# The special doctor-patient relationship

The doctor-patient relationship in endometriosis is distinctive in several ways. While all of the guidelines for any successful partnership apply, there are certain conditions that make an endometriosis patient's relationship with her doctor unique.

*Endometriosis is chronic.* When you are diagnosed as having endometriosis, most often it is the beginning of a long, close working relationship with your doctor. In many cases, you have already been under the doctor's care for months as your symptoms were monitored and finally diagnosed.

You and your doctor both know that the only cure for endometriosis is hysterectomy or menopause. Other treatments may make the symptoms bearable for some patients but they need to be tailored to each woman's life and career.

As a woman with endometriosis, you may undergo one or more surgical procedures, which can add a powerful emotional charge to your interaction with your doctor. No matter what the complexity of the operation, or its outcome, you will call upon your doctor to provide comfort and reassurance to yourself and your family before and after the procedure. You have to feel comfortable in asking for such support and feel confident that your doctor can provide it.

*Endometriosis is intense.* Although you know that your condition is not life-threatening, you have to deal with its painful, debilitating, demoralizing nature. The search for a successful treatment can become an obsession. You'll find that you will look to your doctor for advice in coping with symptoms and the side effects of treatment. This can be emotionally exhausting – for both you and your doctor.

At the same time, you may be in constant pain, be irritable or fatigued. Your doctor, seeing and hearing regularly of your unremitting distress, may feel frustrated and helpless.

Here is a case that illustrates the potential for emotional trauma to both the patient and her doctor. The patient, Mary, was first diagnosed with endometriosis in her early 20s and had eight operations to treat her condition. Still, she continued to suffer terrible pain each month. Finally, at the age of 33, Mary agreed with her doctor that the only treatment left to her was a complete hysterectomy.

After the operation her pain abated for a few months then returned just as strong as before. Mary's doctor suspected that she had a tiny piece of ovary left, which was causing her to continue to ovulate each month. This condition, which occurs in about one per cent of hysterectomies, is considered inoperable because the fragment is almost always too small to be visible to the naked eye (see Chapter 7). The doctor told Mary he could help her only somewhat by prescribing pain relief medication.

Mary was emotionally devastated by the years of unrelenting pain, while the doctor felt a deep sense of failure that even as a last resort the operation had not improved his patient's condition. Still, after talking extensively with her doctor about her condition and options, Mary agreed to take the prescription, which keeps her pain at a manageable level. She continues to trust her doctor and feels that because of his advice and support, she is able to make the best of a difficult situation.

*Endometriosis affects life decisions.* Your condition may have an impact on your decision to have children, your intimate relationships, and the progress of your career. The doctor inevitably becomes involved in decisions on crucial, very personal matters.

For example, a patient who is planning to get married may postpone her wedding until after she completes a six-month course of Danazol because of the possible side effects of the drug. Doctors are called upon to provide counselling on the advisability of such decisions in the light of the stage and possible course of the disease. The doctors' advice is based on a certain amount of guesswork, and the outcome isn't always what they or their patients had hoped for or planned.

Take the example of Joanna, age 22, a patient who started experiencing an intense recurrence of pain eight months after conservative surgery. She was planning her wedding but wanted to wait several years before having children. However, her doctor, after performing laser surgery, suggested that Joanna try to get pregnant quickly, as her disease was progressing at a rapid rate and her symptoms were likely to recur quickly. Joanna trusted her doctor and followed his advice, even though it meant changing her plans to get her career off the ground before starting a family.

Endometriosis patients report that it is essential to find a doctor who understands the physical and emotional impact of the disease and who will provide needed counselling and support. Finding such a doctor can sometimes make the difference between a patient who makes a successful adjustment to emdometriosis, and one who is emotionally defeated by it.

In order to help you develop a solid relationship with your doctor, we have included some basic guidelines for building good communication. These rules apply to any relationship where mutual trust and respect are needed. They are especially important, however, when dealing with the treatment of endometriosis – where you are likely to have a long, intense relationship with your doctor, and in which making important life decisions plays a central part in your treatment process.

The word communication derives from the Latin *communis*, meaning *common*. The goal of doctor-patient communication is to establish a common ground. Some patients – although fewer today than in the past – place their doctor on a pedestal, accepting his or her advice without question. This does not create a 'common ground', the patient just follows instructions whether or not she understands the nature of the disease, the treatment, or its risks.

You should not fall prey to the attitude of blindly obeying your doctor's every suggestion as though it were a command from on high. Instead, ask your doctor questions in order to understand exactly what's wrong with you, how you will be treated, and what the results of each procedure are likely to be.

Reaching this sort of understanding does not happen all at once; it is a process in which both doctor and patient must participate. In brief, the process is as follows: the patient takes a piece of information – such as the symptom of painful intercourse – and transmits this information to the doctor. The doctor receives the information and processes it through his or her own experience and understanding. This can be seen as a sort of translation. For example, the doctor might translate the pain you describe as 'possible involvement of the ligaments at the back of the uterus'. He or she can then act on the belief in that possibility.

This kind of real communication is effective only when all steps of the process are performed by both doctor and patients. You, the patient, must have clear information to begin with, and you must express yourself to your doctor completely, accurately, and in a way that your doctor can understand. Your doctor must in turn receive and process the information in a way that corresponds to your expression.

This all sounds well and good, but what does it mean as a guideline for good communication between doctor and patient in real situations? To answer that question, it is best to break down the suggestions into separate steps.

*The patient must have clear information to begin with.* You must be able to describe your symptoms, know your family history, including any past treatment you or a family member (sister, mother, or grandmother) has had for endometriosis. You should be in touch with your feelings – physical and emotional – concerning your disease and always provide your doctor with clear, correct information. This may mean you have to learn some basic facts about your body and your condition.

*You, the patient, must convert your thoughts and feelings into words the doctor can understand.* This is not easy when the topic is frightening or emotionally charged – such as chronic pain, infertility, or the prospect of surgery – but it must be done. Doctors, for their part, must express their messages in terms you, the patient, will understand. They must find out your level of technical and medical knowledge, and either educate you as necessary for you to understand your condition or explain the situation in simpler terms. Many patients will take it upon themselves to learn about the disease on their own. It is in your best interests to do so. As you are learning, however, feel free to let your doctor know what you do not understand. He or she should either answer your questions or direct you to a source that can.

Effective transmission of a message means the message must 'sink in'. This doesn't always happen in conversation, especially between a doctor and patient – remember the example at the beginning of this chapter of patients watching themselves discuss upcoming surgery. If you are a patient and your doctor has just told you that you may never be able to have children, it's very likely that nothing else the physician says to you for the rest of the visit will 'sink in'. So, instructions on when and how to take medication, information about potentially dangerous or debilitating side effects, and what to do about them will go unheeded.

To avoid this problem, you should always ask to have instructions written down and call your doctor if you have any questions. When one patient, Marta, was taking ampicillin for a lung infection, she experienced a recurrence of the abdominal pain she had been treating with oral contraceptives for months. She asked her doctor what she should make of the pain. The doctor explained that ampicillin decreases the efficacy of oral contraceptives and adjusted Marta's dosage accordingly, so her pain was once again under control.

*You and your doctor must be 'on the same wavelength'.* What does this mean? When you ask your doctor a question to obtain information, he or she should not feel as though you are challenging his or her credibility. By the same token, when a doctor describes a drug's possible side effects, you ought not to feel the physician is doing this to scare you. Remember that the more medical expertise you as a patient have, and the more understanding of your feelings the doctor has, the better the communication process works.

This process sounds simple enough on paper. Keep in mind, though, that, as a patient with endometriosis, you may be frightened, in pain, or intimidated and frustrated by the complexities of this condition. Do all you can to keep these feelings from overwhelming you. Be informed. Ask your doctor for pamphlets or booklets on endometriosis. If you do not understand what your doctor tells you, do not hesitate to ask questions and make suggestions, such as:

- I'm too scared about my operation to absorb what you're saying. Can we talk on the phone later?
- Please define that word
- I don't understand why this procedure is necessary.

If you do not feel you understood what your doctor has told you, you should confirm the message by repeating it back:

• So you feel that the best treatment would be to take Danazol for six months, followed by conservative surgery?

If the doctor is not sure that you have grasped the full meaning of a diagnosis or suggested treatment, he or she may ask you questions such as:

• What other questions do you have about laser laparoscopy?
• Is it clear that Danazol has several side effects that may be unpleasant, but that they are not dangerous?
• Will you be able to take a month off from your job to recover from surgery?

# Final tips for becoming a better patient

*Ask informed questions.* You need to know basic things about how your body works and what endometriosis does to it if you want to know how to best manage your condition. You should be able to ask your doctor the following:

• How will the diagnosis take place?
• What kinds of medications are available? What are the side effects? Which side effects are benign (not serious), which could be dangerous? How will I feel when I am on the medication?
• What else besides drugs and surgery may help my condition? Would a different diet or a programme of exercise make a difference in the progress of treatment? How can I control the pain?
• How will I feel after the laparoscopy? Are there things I can do to relieve any pain or discomfort?
• How long will I be incapacitated after the surgery? What are the possible complications?

Patients will find that the more *informed, specific* questions they are able to ask about their endometriosis, the more they will be able to learn from their doctor. While this may not help with the progress of their treatment, it will add to their sense of well-being and to their doctor's. For example, Lisa was a patient who had endured such terrible pain from endometriosis that her doctor finally suggested that, at the age of 30, she have a complete hysterectomy. Lisa did not seek a second opinion (even though her doctor urged her to) and went ahead with the procedure without understanding how a hysterectomy would affect her physically and emotionally. Later she suffered severe depression. It took years of psychotherapy for Lisa to work out her hurt and anger over the devastating effects of her cure.

*Write things down.* In managing a condition as complex as endometriosis, you should get in the habit of keeping important information on paper: questions for your doctor, details of your family history, records of symptoms, a menstrual diary, dates of any surgery, length and outcome of drug treatments, etc. Organize this information carefully and have it readily accessible. Of course, your doctor will keep records of most of this medical data, but you never know when you may need to have your own information at your fingertips.

The questionnaire below is one that I give to all patients with known or suspected endometriosis. I encourage them to keep a copy of their own and to maintain up-to-date, accurate records as their condition changes. The chart is most useful if you to answer the questions as honestly and completely as possible.

*Try to get the support of friends and family.* Because the disease affects their daily lives, most patients find that their ability to handle endometriosis depends on the support of people close to them. You will probably find that you have a more positive relationship with your doctor and are able to cope better if you tell people who are close to you about your condition, how it's being treated, and how endometriosis and its treatment are likely to affect your life. If you feel that the disease poses a serious threat

50

Name:

Age:

Number of Pregnancies:

Age periods began:

Duration of period:

Pain before period? yes ☐ no ☐

Pain with period? yes ☐ no ☐

Pain with ovulation? yes ☐ no ☐

Duration of pain:

Site of pain (right or left side?):     Lasting

Pain with intercourse? yes ☐ no ☐ how long?

Pain with bowel movement? yes ☐ no ☐

Bleeding from rectum? yes ☐ no ☐

Pain with urination? yes ☐ no ☐

Bleeding between periods? yes ☐ no ☐

Heavy periods? yes ☐ no ☐

Irregular periods? yes ☐ no ☐

Skipped periods? yes ☐ no ☐

Fever? yes ☐ no ☐

Enlarged lymph glands? yes ☐ no ☐

Flulike symptoms (lethargy,
   muscle aches)? yes ☐ no ☐

Fatigue? yes ☐ no ☐

Backache? yes ☐ no ☐

Constipation? yes ☐ no ☐

Diarrhoea? yes ☐ no ☐

to your relationship with your husband or lover, you may want to see a marriage counsellor or sex therapist together to talk about the disease's disruptive effects on your lives. Many of my patients have taken this step.

*Keep your expectations realistic.* Although knowledge about endometriosis is growing, many patients still expect or hope for a quick, simple cure. They become angry and frustrated with their doctor when this doesn't happen. Sometimes they even change their medication schedules or stop taking their prescribed drugs without telling their doctor, which can be dangerous and lead to a worsening of their condition.

A colleague of mine told me of a patient who didn't like the side effects of Danazol, so she stopped taking her medication after two months. Her pain did not return so she never saw her doctor again – that is, until she had to have emergency surgery for a ruptured cyst.

As we've said before, the more you learn about endometriosis, the more 'common ground' you share with your doctor. As a result, you'll be better able to share a realistic understanding of the seriousness of your condition, how it is being treated, and your prospects for the future.

As a final word on this subject, we want to remind you that neither you nor your doctor should expect the worst. Keep an optimistic attitude. Many patients improve under treatment more than their doctors expect. There's no reason not to hope for the best – relief from pain or the ability to have children – and to work with the doctor to bring about the best possible result.

# Chapter 3

# WHAT CAUSES ENDOMETRIOSIS?

My main question to you is, what causes endometriosis? I have seen seven doctors and had two laparoscopies. Every doctor I asked said that there are a couple of theories. But they don't tell me what the theories are. Or they say they don't really know.

*A 25-year-old patient*

One of the most baffling things about endometriosis is that no one knows how it starts – how or why a substance resembling the lining of the uterus and having a specific function within that organ grows in other parts of the body where it is clearly not needed. This is one of the first questions most patients ask me, and I can respond only by telling them the theories of what *may* cause endometriosis. If doctors could tell their patients why it occurs, we would certainly be a lot closer to understanding how to prevent and treat the condition.

Over the years, doctors have put forth their share of theories on the causes of endometriosis. However, whether or not they had data to back these theories suggested in the past – and even those considered plausible today – they make endometriosis sound like a strange and mysterious condition indeed.

In this chapter we shall briefly trace the development of the three principal theories which attempt to explain the cause of endometriosis.

The first written record we have of a scientist venturing to suggest a possible cause of endometriosis comes from the German doctor Von Recklinghausen. In 1895 this doctor posited that the masses of tissue he could feel adhering to the pelvic organs of his female patients actually were the remnants of 'an embryologic urological system' – the method of waste disposal used in the foetal state. This was known as the theory of Wolffian duct rest, and attracted quite a bit of notoriety in the medical community. However, its influence was short-lived.

The theory did influence the work of another doctor who also was concerned about the abdominal pain several of his patients were experiencing. A year later a British scientist by the name of Cullen was able, through manual pelvic examination of his female patients, to detect what he believed to be masses of tissue on their ovaries and fallopian tubes. These findings led him to suggest, in a conclusion similar to Dr Von Recklinghausen's, that the growths were actually the remains of the primitive structures from which these organs grew in their embryonic state. This theory did not last long, either.

Neither scientist used the word endometriosis; nor do their writings suggest that they saw any connection between the growths and the endometrium, or lining of the uterus. These early theories make interesting – and somewhat amusing – historical reading, but as a patient trying to understand the cause of your endometriosis, you are best off putting them aside.

A much more probable – and plausible – suggestion for the cause of endometriosis was put forth just after the turn of the century by two researchers named Ivanoff and Meyer. They suggested that cell changes on the surfaces of organ tissue – not mysterious primitive growths on the female urologic and reproductive organs – caused the painful, debilitating masses in the abdominal cavity that tormented their female patients. They suggested that under 'correct stimulation' the cells of the surface of the reproductive organs underwent a change that allowed the abnormal growths to form and grow.

While Ivanoff and Meyer's theory went no further in trying to explain exactly what these cell changes were, what prompted them, and why they occurred in some women and not in others, the idea made sense – and forms the basis of one of today's three main theories of what causes endometriosis.

Most scientists nowadays accept at least one of the three 'classic' theories outlined below as a probable cause of endometriosis. I find that there are both useful and baffling elements in each of the three theories.

# Transplantation theory

Medical researcher John Sampson is credited with being the first to use the term endometriosis. He applied it in 1921 to a condition in which, as he described it, the lining of the uterus backs up and out of the fallopian tubes and into the abdominal cavity, adhering to the pelvic organs. This theory won immediate widespread acceptance as a likely cause of the painful disorder, which otherwise was unexplained.

Actually, Sampson's theory has held up rather well under the test of time. Studies today show that women who have obstructions of the lower genital tract that might cause menstrual fluid to 'back up', such as vaginal and uterine infections, have higher rates of endometriosis than the general population of women.

However, a study conducted as recently as 1984 has cast doubt on Sampson's theory. Researchers at the University of North Carolina discovered that 90 per cent of 52 women with functioning fallopian tubes showed some back up of endometrial fluid – known as retrograde bleeding (see figure 1) – during menstruation. If this is so, the researchers – and the rest of the medical community – wondered, why doesn't 90 per cent of the population of women also develop endometriosis?

Several other recent studies have supported this finding and raised the same question, and in 1986 the same research team reinforced their own original findings by showing that 90 per cent of a group of 250 women who had tubal ligations had some retrograde bleeding during menstruation – but not one had endometriosis.

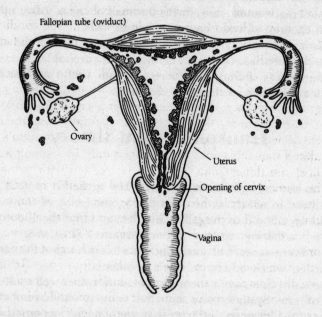

Fallopian tube (oviduct)

Ovary

Uterus

Opening of cervix

Vagina

*Figure 2* Retrograde bleeding through the fallopian tubes.

In addition, studies on female monkeys have found that when the uterus is surgically turned upside down, so that the cervix – the neck of the uterus that normally extends down into the vagina – faces upward and menstrual fluid flows into the abdominal cavity, only 60 per cent of the monkeys developed endometriosis.

What do these findings tell us? That Sampson's theory goes only part of the way in explaining the cause of endometriosis. Clinical observations do indeed suggest that some women develop the condition as a direct result of retrograde bleeding. But why the back up of fluid forms implants in some women and not in others remains a mystery. The monkey experiment invalidates the claim that many doctors have made that it's the *amount* of fluid that flows out of the uterus that determines whether a woman will develop endometriosis. Retrograde bleeding may indeed play some role in causing the condition, but the recent experiments show that there must be other factors at work as well.

Sampson's theory also fails to explain why some patients develop endometriosis in sites distant from the uterus, such as the groin, armpits, lungs, even the nasal passages. Although such cases are rare, they have been carefully documented. Another scientist studying the disorder back in Sampson's day postulated that this could be explained only by looking at the condition on the cellular level.

The human body transports material – mainly oxygen and nutrients to nourish the cells – through two systems: the circulatory and the lymphatic. The former circulates blood; the latter serves basically to cleanse our internal organs, removing impurities and concentrating them at sites throughout the body, called lymph nodes, from which they are disposed of. In 1927, a medical researcher named Halban made the suggestion that both of these systems could transport cells from the lining of the uterus to other parts of the body in women with endometriosis. And since no one else at the time could explain how the endometrial implants might end up outside the endometrial cavity – in the lungs or nasal passages, for example – Halban's theory gained credibility.

The theory remains a credible basis for explaining the presence of endometriosis in parts of the body distant from the uterus. However, it suffers from the same shortcomings as Sampson's transplantation theory, in that it fails to explain why the condition occurs in some women and not in others. Most women have retrograde bleeding during their periods, and all have blood and lymph fluid circulating through their bodies continuously.

Clearly, other facts must play a part in causing endometriosis.

# Metaplastic theory

The term *metaplasia* means a change in the characteristics of cells. The idea of changes at the cellular level leading to endometriosis intrigued another contemporary of Sampson's, a researcher by the name of Meyer. He suggested that repeated irritation of the cells of the lining of the abdominal cavity – for example, due to a recurring infection – could cause the cell changes that lead to endometriosis.

Although Meyer did not back up his theory with clinical observations, recent findings about who gets endometriosis have tended to confirm his ideas. For example, in the two known cases of endometriosis in men, both were taking high doses of the female hormone oestrogen, which affects the characteristics of cells, particularly in men.

In addition, women with primary amenorrhoea (cessation of their menstrual periods) and those whose mothers took the hormone diethylstilbesterol (DES) while they were pregnant seem to have higher rates of endometriosis than the general population of women, according to several recent studies.

In both of these conditions, higher than normal levels of the hormone oestrogen are present in the abdominal cavity. If Meyer's theory is correct, these increased hormonal levels are responsible for the development of endometriosis.

Scientists are still studying the possible effects of hormonal changes on the cells of the lining of the abdominal cavity. At the moment it is an area of complex and intense research. Doctors hope to discover the link between cell changes that are caused by infections, medication, and other disturbances, and the development of endometriosis.

At the same time, other researchers are examining the last of the three classic theories attempting to explain the cause of the condition.

# Induction theory

This theory again suggests that changes at the level of the cell are responsible for endometriosis. This time, however, scientists suggest chemical substances introduced from the outside cause the changes that lead to the condition.

In the latter part of the nineteenth century, the researcher Lavendar postulated that cells outside the uterus could be transformed to resemble endometrial cells if they were chemically stimulated. Scientific experimentation has not completely supported – or even fully explained – this somewhat bizarre theory. But researchers have not yet let go of the possibility that a chemical introduced from outside the body and acting at the cellular level may in some way be responsible for the development of endometriosis. For example, some doctors have attempted to determine whether women who have had Caesarean sections or other abdominal surgery have a higher incidence of endometriosis than the general population of women.

So far, however, the results of such studies have been inconclusive. Though such possibilities are intriguing and further research into them is important, I believe that the explanation of the cause of the condition lies in other directions.

A critical look at the three classical theories of the cause of endometriosis shows that all fall short of explaining to women with the condition why they have it and other women don't. As a result, the most recent – and, I believe, most exciting – research has started to look into completely different possible causes.

# The immune system

Many scientists today believe that the body's immune mechanism is altered in important ways in women with endometriosis, allowing implantation of tissue in parts of the body other than where they are normally found to take place in those women predisposed to the condition. In other words, these researchers suggest, some women are born with a deficient immune system that in some way makes them more prone to developing endometriosis.

This theory does not mean that all women so disposed to endometriosis will get it. It only suggests that their risk is greater than normal. Nor does it mean that these women are more susceptible to any other sort of infection, because this type of immune deficiency is not related to the prevention of infection.

The fact that a tendency to develop endometriosis appears to be inherited supports this immune-deficiency theory. Studies have shown that a woman whose close relative (mother, grandmother, sister, daughter) has endometriosis is up to seven times more likely than the average woman to develop it herself.

More and more scientists studying endometriosis today believe that the condition is caused by what's known as an *auto-immune deficiency*. With this condition the body is unable to defend itself from a threat from within.

If this theory ever proves true, the facts would form the 'missing link' in completing Sampson's retrograde bleeding theory. As we have suggested, if retrograde bleeding occurs in most women, then most of them must also have a built-in mechanism that rejects endometrial fluid outside the uterus – otherwise most women would develop endometriosis. In women who do get the condition, the theory goes, this mechanism either does not work at all or does an inadequate job.

Scientists believe that some of the major life-threatening diseases of our times may be caused by an auto-immune deficiency: diabetes, multiple sclerosis, arthritis, cancer, and, most obviously, AIDS. This makes the quest to find ways to treat and prevent these diseases a very important area in medical research. For example, cancer researchers have discovered that most people produce some cancer cells, which are destroyed by our immune systems.

Researchers looking for ways to prevent and treat endometriosis believe that the same principle applies to women with the condition: like the majority of women, they have retrograde bleeding, but the menstrual fluid, instead of being rejected outside the uterus by an auto-immune response, is allowed to adhere to other parts of the body. A deficiency in the immune systems of these women prevents them from rejecting the endometrial cells.

Scientists studying endometriosis hope that they will one day develop a vaccine to prevent the condition in women whose systems don't naturally have the ability to reject the lining of the uterus outside that organ. Patients often ask me about the possibility of such a development; however, the latest medical literature indicates that it is not likely within the next several years.

A word or two is needed at this point on some of the factors which we know do *not* cause endometriosis. I find that I am constantly assuring my patients that various factors, both within and beyond their control, are not responsible for their disease.

Endometriosis is a very stressful condition for most women. If the pain isn't enough to throw them off their emotional balance, the accompanying infertility – or at least worry over its possibility in the future – reduces the quality of life for even the most stable, otherwise contented women. One woman wrote to me after reading an interview published in a magazine: '[After surgery] I was still in so much pain, one time I wanted to just kill myself to escape the pain. My doctor mentioned hysterectomy and that seemed out of the question at the age of 20 . . . It's so hard at times I could just scream.'

Perhaps because many women with endometriosis have such a stressed response to their condition, some doctors have suggested that stress *causes* endometriosis. If these women would just relax, these doctors say – about their careers, their painful periods, possible infertility – their symptoms would disappear.

These doctors are making a big mistake and looking at the wrong culprit. Stress is a popular scapegoat these days. It is blamed for causing many of our modern woes – from impotence to the common cold. While there certainly is evidence that many people would be a lot healthier if they could become more relaxed, it is certain that endometriosis is one condition for which there's absolutely no evidence of a connection to stress. Stress does not cause endometriosis. I've always found that women who get the disease range in their ability to take life easy in the same way as the general population of both women *and* men.

Still, some doctors try to uphold the myth of stress causing endometriosis by pointing out that the majority of women who seek treatment for the condition are those our society tends to label as the most highly stressed – professional, white, well-educated 'career' women who are delaying having children until their mid-thirties or even later. In fact, you may even have heard endometriosis referred to as the 'career woman's disease'.

The fact – overlooked by these doctors – is that so-called 'career' women are simply more likely than less well-educated, non-professional, non-white women to seek medical attention for *any* condition. To prove the point, recent research is showing that endometriosis is just as common among non-white, non-working women of low socioeconomic status. These women are simply less likely than other women to seek treatment.

Another popular myth about endometriosis is that delayed childbearing 'causes' the condition. We would not want to venture to guess the number of women whose doctors have told them, 'This never would have happened if you hadn't waited so long to start a family.' If your doctor conveys this message to you, I would recommend that you start looking for another doctor right away.

Delayed childbearing allows the condition to progress more quickly in women *already predisposed to develop it*, simply because it cannot progress, due to hormonal alterations and changes in the uterine lining, during the nine months a woman is pregnant. One patient I know had four children after she was diagnosed as having endometriosis. Each time she became pregnant, her symptoms diminished or disappeared for the nine months until she gave birth. However, they returned again within three months of her delivery.

## WHAT CAUSES ENDOMETRIOSIS?

As a doctor, I would love to be able to tell every patient with endometriosis exactly how she developed the condition. But for now, that's usually just not possible. However, a woman *can* gain a fairly accurate idea of how serious her case is, and what her condition may mean in terms of her future fertility. The system for determining these facts is outlined in the next chapter.

# Chapter 4

# A CLASSIFICATION SYSTEM

When a woman is diagnosed as having endometriosis, her first question to her doctor is likely to be, 'How bad is it?' Until recently, doctors felt frustrated that they could not give their endometriosis patients a very satisfactory answer to that question. Today, more and more doctors are able to tell their patients quite accurately how serious their condition is, as well as its likely outcome. Although this doesn't reduce their symptoms, it does make their condition much easier to handle emotionally.

Until 1985, doctors used three main systems to classify the disease. Obviously, this made things confusing for the doctor – not to mention the patient – and made communication about the condition within the medical community very difficult. Doctors exchanging information about their patients had no basis for comparing the relative severities of various patients, which made it almost impossible for them to have any discussion of treatments.

One system was developed by Robert Kistner, MD, a prominent research scientist at Harvard Medical School in the USA. The second had been created in the 1970s by the American Fertility Society, an organization of medical specialists studying and promoting fertility. It was used only erratically. The third and most widely used, also developed in

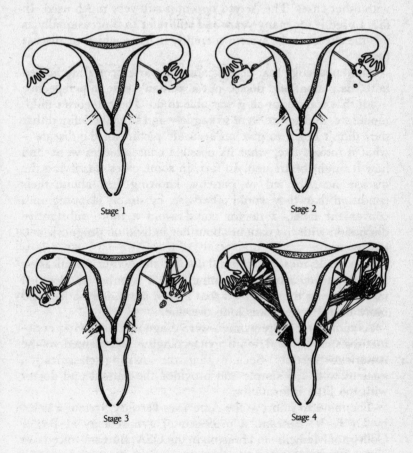

*Figure 3*   The advance of endometriosis on the ovaries and fallopian tubes.

the 1970s, was known as the Acosta system. Using it, doctors could classify a case of endometriosis as mild, moderate, or severe, a classification that at least gave the patient a word to describe what she was experiencing and a basis of comparison with other cases. The Acosta system is still very much used. In fact I used it for many years and still refer to it occasionally as it is the closest to the system currently in use – which we discuss below.

The knowledge that classification imparted certainly helped both the patient and doctor put a woman's case in perspective – but that was about all it was able to do. The categories mild, moderate, and severe were so vaguely and broadly defined that they didn't begin to give an accurate picture of the disease – what it looked like, what its possible consequences were, and how it might be treated. In fact, in some cases classifying the disease actually led to patients knowing less about their condition than they would otherwise; by simply slapping on a convenient label, a doctor could avoid a more substantive discussion with the patient about her individual prognosis and treatment.

As a result, most patients did not find the Acosta classification system particularly enlightening and a number of doctors, myself among them, agreed that a new, more descriptive, and more useful system was long overdue.

As more and more women were diagnosed as having endometriosis, more and more gynaecologists complained to the American Fertility Society that the existing classification systems were too simple and provided the patient and doctor with too little information.

The move to improve the American Fertility System was led by Dr E. V. Butram, a professor of gynaecology at Baylor College of Medicine in Houston in the USA. Butram voiced two main complaints; that the current systems did not promote a clear picture of what the patient's condition meant in terms of her fertility, and that they provided almost no information that could be applied to research. Doctors wanted to classify patients in a way that would enable them to start amassing a data bank that would tell them who was getting the disease, what the typical case was like and, from that information, a picture of what treatments were and were not working.

In 1985 the American Fertility Society responded to these

many requests by issuing an updated version of its classification system. The new system, which today is in much wider use than any of the old ones, is superior in several ways.

Instead of three levels of severity, it has four – minimal, mild, moderate, and severe. The main advantage of the addition of a fourth (and least severe) category is that it allows doctors to diagnose and classify cases at earlier stages, when treatment of the condition is almost always easier and less costly.

In addition, the system also allows doctors to tell patients at each stage the approximate number, size, and location of implants on each side of their body. The old systems did not even tell the patient whether endometriosis was affecting one or both sides. Therefore, a patient could be classified as severe, with implants completely covering one ovary and fallopian tube, yet find to her own and her doctor's surprise that she was able to become pregnant. On the other hand, a patient classified as moderate, with implants only partially covering each of her ovaries and fallopian tubes, might at first think that her case is not serious and later discover that she is irreparably infertile.

The old system listed six possible sites for endometriosis: the ovaries, fallopian tubes, bladder, bowel, appendix, and the broad ligaments in the back of the abdominal cavity known as the peritoneum. To these the new system added a seventh, the cul-de-sac, an area just under and behind the uterus. This turns out to be a very common site of endometriosis, with implants there affecting 30 to 40 per cent of patients and, for most of them, causing the greatest amount of pain because the area is inaccessible, yet attached to the uterus.

A final improvement of the new classification system over the old ones is that it allows doctors to describe the implants on the ovaries, peritoneum, and fallopian tubes as either 'filmy' or 'dense' and 'superficial' or 'deep'. In addition to helping patients, the addition of such descriptions educates doctors by broadening their understanding of what endometriosis actually looks like.

The chart on pp 68–69 shows the new American Fertility Society

# ENDOMETRIOSIS

**THE AMERICAN FERTILITY SOCIETY
REVISED CLASSIFICATION OF ENDOMETRIOSIS**

Patient's Name _____ Date _____

Stage I   (Minimal)  · 1-5
Stage II  (Mild)     · 6-15        Laparoscopy _____ Laparotomy _____ Photography _____
Stage III (Moderate) · 16-40       Recommended Treatment _____
Stage IV  (Severe)   · >40         _____
Total _____                      Prognosis _____

| | ENDOMETRIOSIS | <1cm | 1-3cm | >3cm |
|---|---|---|---|---|
| **PERITONEUM** | Superficial | 1 | 2 | 4 |
| | Deep | 2 | 4 | 6 |
| **OVARY** | R  Superficial | 1 | 2 | 4 |
| | Deep | 4 | 16 | 20 |
| | L  Superficial | 1 | 2 | 4 |
| | Deep | 4 | 16 | 20 |

| | POSTERIOR CULDESAC OBLITERATION | Partial | | Complete | |
|---|---|---|---|---|---|
| | | 4 | | 40 | |

| | ADHESIONS | <1/3 Enclosure | 1/3-2/3 Enclosure | >2/3 Enclosure |
|---|---|---|---|---|
| **OVARY** | R  Filmy | 1 | 2 | 4 |
| | Dense | 4 | 8 | 16 |
| | L  Filmy | 1 | 2 | 4 |
| | Dense | 4 | 8 | 16 |
| **TUBE** | R  Filmy | 1 | 2 | 4 |
| | Dense | 4* | 8* | 16 |
| | L  Filmy | 1 | 2 | 4 |
| | Dense | 4* | 8* | 16 |

*If the fimbriated end of the fallopian tube is completely enclosed, change the point assignment to 16.

Additional Endometriosis: _____        Associated Pathology: _____
_____        _____
_____        _____

**To Be Used with Normal
Tubes and Ovaries**

L                                R

**To Be Used with Abnormal
Tubes and/or Ovaries**

L                                R

*Chart 1*

68

# A CLASSIFICATION SYSTEM

**EXAMPLES & GUIDELINES**

| STAGE I (MINIMAL) | STAGE II (MILD) | STAGE III (MODERATE) |
|---|---|---|

**STAGE I (MINIMAL)**

PERITONEUM
Superficial Endo – 1-3cm · 2
R. OVARY
Superficial Endo – < 1cm · 1
Filmy Adhesions – < 1/3 · 1
TOTAL POINTS 4

**STAGE II (MILD)**

PERITONEUM
Deep Endo – > 3cm · 6
R. OVARY
Superficial Endo – < 1cm · 1
Filmy Adhesions – < 1/3 · 1
L. OVARY
Superficial Endo – < 1cm · 1
TOTAL POINTS 9

**STAGE III (MODERATE)**

PERITONEUM
Deep Endo – > 3cm · 6
CULDESAC
Partial Obliteration · 4
L. OVARY
Deep Endo – 1-3cm · 16
TOTAL POINTS 26

| STAGE III (MODERATE) | STAGE IV (SEVERE) | STAGE IV (SEVERE) |
|---|---|---|

**STAGE III (MODERATE)**

PERITONEUM
Superficial Endo – > 3cm · 4
R. TUBE
Filmy Adhesions – < 1/3 · 1
R. OVARY
Filmy Adhesions – < 1/3 · 1
L. TUBE
Dense Adhesions – < 1/3 · 16*
L. OVARY
Deep Endo – < 1 cm · 4
Dense Adhesions – < 1/3 · 4
TOTAL POINTS 30

**STAGE IV (SEVERE)**

PERITONEUM
Superficial Endo – > 3cm · 4
L. OVARY
Deep Endo – 1-3cm · 32**
Dense Adhesions – < 1/3 · 8**
L. TUBE
Dense Adhesions – < 1/3 · 8**
TOTAL POINTS 52

**STAGE IV (SEVERE)**

PERITONEUM
Deep Endo – > 3cm · 6
CULDESAC
Complete Obliteration · 40
R. OVARY
Deep Endo – 1-3cm · 16
Dense Adhesions – < 1/3 · 4
L. TUBE
Dense Adhesions – > 2/3 · 16
L. OVARY
Deep Endo – 1-3cm · 16
Dense Adhesions – > 2/3 · 16
TOTAL POINTS 114

*Point assignment changed to 16
**Point assignment doubled

Determination of the stage or degree of endometrial involvement is based on a weighted point system. Distribution of points has been arbitrarily determined and may require further revision or refinement as knowledge of the disease increases.

To ensure complete evaluation, inspection of the pelvis in a clockwise or counterclockwise fashion is encouraged. Number, size and location of endometrial implants, plaques, endometriomas and/or adhesions are noted. For example, five separate 0.5cm superficial implants on the peritoneum (2.5 cm total) would be assigned 2 points. (The surface of the uterus should be considered peritoneum.) The severity of the endometriosis or adhesions should be assigned the highest score only for peritoneum, ovary, tube or culdesac. For example, a 4cm superficial and a 2cm deep implant of the peritoneum should be given a score of 6 (not 8). A 4cm deep endometrioma of the ovary associated with more than 3cm of superficial disease should be scored 20 (not 24).

In those patients with only one adnexa, points applied to disease of the remaining tube and ovary should be multiplied by two. **Points assigned may be circled and totaled. Aggregation of points indicates stage of disease (minimal, mild, moderate, or severe).

The presence of endometriosis of the bowel, urinary tract, fallopian tube, vagina, cervix, skin etc., should be documented under "additional endometriosis." Other pathology such as tubal occlusion, leiomyomata, uterine anomaly, etc., should be documented under "associated pathology." All pathology should be depicted as specifically as possible on the sketch of pelvic organs, and means of observation (laparoscopy or laparotomy) should be noted.

*Chart 2*

69

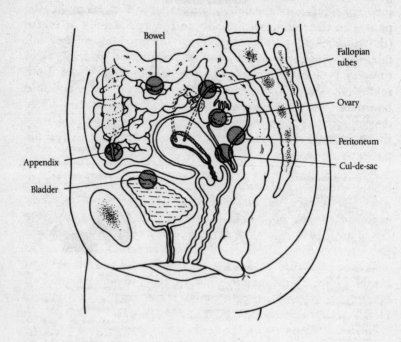

*Figure 4* The usual sites of endometriosis.

system of classification for endometriosis, which has been adopted as the international standard. Although British gynaecologists use the AFS system, they do not usually use this chart. It has been included here to show how the system works.

The first page of the chart allows the doctor to indicate the number and size of each implant or cluster of implants on the peritoneum and cul-de-sac and each tube and ovary, and whether the adhesions are 'filmy' or 'dense' and whether the implants are 'superficial' or 'deep'. Thus the doctor assigns the adhesion or implant the designated number of points.

The drawings on the second page of the classification form

give the doctor guidelines for evaluating each case and taking into consideration special circumstances. For example, the patient in the middle of the bottom row is classified as severe (the number of points assigned to the growths on her left fallopian tube and ovary is doubled because the woman's right tube and ovary either are not functioning or have been removed). Notice, however, that the patient's point total would be under forty if the system just took into account the development of the condition on one side of her body. Under the old system such special considerations were not part of the patient's evaluation.

Most doctors strongly recommend that a patient suspected of having the disorder have a laparoscopy, an operation in which a small incision is made just above the navel to allow examination of the abdominal cavity. (For a complete description of the procedure, see Chapter 5.) Only with this procedure can the doctor really see the extent of the disease as well as the location of the major implants. As you should now be able to see, this information is crucial in planning with your doctor the type of surgical and/or drug treatment you will receive.

Since both the new and the old classification systems use the terms mild, moderate, and severe to classify the stages of endometriosis (although, as we mentioned, the new system starts off with the classification minimal), it is crucial that you, as the patient, make sure that you and your doctor are using the same system to classify your disease. Failure to do so can result in confusion about the severity of your case. A case history, involving the patient of a doctor I know, illustrates the importance of making this distinction.

Maria, a woman in her early twenties with a five-year-old daughter, had been having severe abdominal pain during her periods for three years. More recently, she had been experiencing pain during intercourse. In late 1985 she described her symptoms to her gynaecologist, who immediately suspected endometriosis. He performed a pelvic examination in his office, and told Maria that she was suffering from stage two of the disease. He suggested drug therapy with Danazol (danol). Before Maria could start the treatment, however, she discovered that she was pregnant.

Maria's symptoms diminished during her pregnancy to the point where she very rarely felt pain. Within three months after giving birth, however, she again started experiencing severe pain during intercourse and around the time of her period.

This time she visited a different gynaecologist, who saw from her medical records that she had stage two endometriosis. 'That's a mild case,' the doctor informed her. 'I wouldn't say you need Danazol treatment at this point. Come back to me in six months if you're still feeling pain.'

As you can imagine, the next six months were agony for Maria. She spent the three or four days a month around her period in bed, doubled up in pain. During this time sex was out of the question.

Finally, Maria visited a third gynaecologist who, when Maria described her severe symptoms, scheduled her to come in for a laparoscopy the next day. The operation found extensive growths on her cul-de-sac, ovaries, and fallopian tubes. The doctor removed four large implants and recommended six months of treatment with Danazol to shrink the remaining growths. Using the newly introduced classification system, he assigned the case a score of 36 on the point scale, which classified it as stage three. Under the new classification system this was considered a 'moderate' case.

Looking over Maria's medical history, the doctor was mystified to find that only a few months earlier her case had been classified as 'mild'. He found it hard to believe that her condition had progressed so quickly in such a short time.

What neither he nor Maria realized was that the doctor she'd visited when her symptoms returned after her pregnancy had neglected to find out whether her previous diagnosis had been made under the old or the new system. By wrongly assuming her first doctor had been using the *new* system, the second doctor had diagnosed Maria's case as 'mild'. Actually she was far worse off, having nearly a severe case under the new system.

The case illustrates how these sorts of misunderstandings are not merely academic. Maria and other patients like her can be spared months, even years, of pain if doctors take the trouble to make certain that everyone involved with a case follows the updated and more detailed classification system.

The case also illustrates the importance of performing a laparoscopy to diagnose every case of endometriosis (again see Chapter 5). Had Maria's second doctor followed the procedure it would have immediately become clear that Maria's case, even if it *had* been mild before her pregnancy, had worsened to the point where she needed immediate treatment through a combination of surgery and drugs. This is why I can't stress enough the importance of a laparoscopy as a standard part of the diagnosis of endometriosis.

There is another advantage of the updated classification system and its widespread use in diagnosing and treating endometriosis patients. Using the system creates a framework within which doctors can get a clearer idea of how many women are getting the disease, at what stage doctors are diagnosing cases, and what methods are being successfully used to treat them.

Gradually, information is emerging on the most common sites for implants, the growing number of patients whose cases are being diagnosed in earlier stages, and the most – and least – successful treatments at each stage. We can look at another case history, again of a patient of a colleague of mine, to illustrate how the system can work.

Margaret was in her late twenties when she first noticed pain around the time of her period. She ignored it for almost a year, until her annual check-up with her gynaecologist, when she mentioned both the pain and her surprise that she was not pregnant. As a devout Catholic, Margaret did not practise birth control, and she had given birth to three babies in the first four years of her marriage. But her youngest child was now almost three – and Margaret was puzzled over the sudden unexplained change in her fertility. Although she said she only felt 'twinges of pain' a few days out of each month – and not necessarily before or during her period – and occasionally during intercourse or a bowel movement, her doctor decided to perform a laparoscopy.

The operation revealed endometrial implants completely covering one of Margaret's ovaries and fallopian tubes, with somewhat less, but still extensive growth on the other side, as well as smaller implants on her cul-de-sac and bowel – in all, enough to classify her case as stage four or 'severe'. Her doctor removed what she could surgically and put Margaret on a nine-month course of Danazol. The patient's reaction to the drug treatment was so negative – weight gain of 30 pounds, deepening of her voice, profuse growth of facial hair, severe bouts of depression and acne – that she begged to be taken off the treatment after only three months.

Despite Margaret's pain, the doctor hesitated. She knew that Margaret wanted more children and wasn't sure that her treatment would shrink the growths enough at this point to allow a reasonable chance for a pregnancy to occur. But by looking over the patient's medical records the doctor was reminded that the growths had invaded one ovary and fallopian tube much more than the other. This meant that it was likely that the less affected side might by now be free enough of implants to allow a reasonable chance of pregnancy.

Moreover, because of her familiarity with the current literature on endometriosis, Margaret's doctor was aware that in a significant percentage of stage three cases treated with surgery followed by Danazol for six to nine months, the patient was able to achieve a pregnancy.

Weighing all these factors, Margaret and her doctor made the decision to take her off the Danazol treatment at the end of five months. To their joy, Margaret discovered that she was pregnant only three months later.

The use of a classification system in treating endometriosis should not obscure the fact that every case of the condition is different. As in treating any medical disorder, what works for one patient has no guarantee of working for another, even though the two may have nearly identical symptoms. But the

doctors and patients should take advantage and use the system
for what it is: a valuable tool for classifying the stages of an often
baffling disorder.

# Chapter 5

# DIAGNOSING ENDOMETRIOSIS

I had resigned myself to the fact that I would *always* be sterile, have 13 to 15-day menstrual periods, transient iron deficiency, anaemia from flooding, sleepless nights from painful menstrual cramps and cyclic bleeding from my urinary tract . . . [My doctor] kept saying I had an infection. Later he said it was kidney stones. When I realized that the bleeding was always at the end of my menstrual period, I knew without a doubt what I had.

*A 34-year-old patient*

The woman whose letter is reprinted above did not have a urinary tract infection or kidney stones, but a severe case of endometriosis, with eight implants and an adhesion wrapped around the bladder. The symptoms she presented – and the action her doctor took until *she* learned the facts and forced them into action – point out the vital importance of getting a definitive diagnosis of endometriosis.

The so-called classic symptoms of the condition are pain during menstruation (dysmenorrhoea), painful intercourse (dyspareunia), and infertility. The majority of patients experience at least one of them during the course of their disease. None of these symptoms – or any of the others – are life-threatening. However, all of them can have serious negative effects on the *quality* of your life.

There are other complications as well for both endometriosis patients and their doctors. For one thing, all three of these symptoms are vague, highly subjective, and often difficult to measure. They can also be the symptoms of many other gynaecological disorders, from pelvic inflammatory disease to ovarian cancer. And some women experience pain and infertility not as the result of any clearly determined physiological disorder.

The best way to illustrate the difficulty in diagnosing endometriosis – and to help explain why so many cases go undiagnosed and untreated for years – is to reprint part of a letter I received from a woman:

> I started having a dull aching on my left side, by the ovary. It came and went and didn't seem to be associated with my period. I just more or less went on with it. I had never heard of endometriosis, let alone the symptoms. I then started having an irritating discharge. It would also come and go. I also started spotting [between periods]. The aching persisted and seemed to get worse with each day, to the point where it would drive me crazy. I went to my family doctor. The ache was so bad it was hard to move and sit. He did a pelvic exam and came to the conclusion it was PID. He gave me [two prescriptions for pain and antibiotics] . . . Ten days later the pain was worse and I was still bleeding heavily. My husband took me to the emergency room and the doctor on call believed I had a tubular [ectopic] pregnancy. He said he felt a small lump of some kind and ordered ultrasound. The radiologist believed I had an ovarian cyst. The doctor ordered a pregnancy test and the results came back negative. He went off duty and another doctor came on who came to the conclusion that it was PID. He gave me prescriptions for pain and very strong antibiotics. I followed up with an appointment with a specialist. He did a pelvic [examination] and also felt the lump. He saw I was in a lot of pain and said he didn't know what was wrong with me, and suggested surgery to see.

When a woman complains to her gynaecologist of pain – painful periods, for example – how is the doctor to know, except through what she reports, how bad the pain really is and what might be causing it? After all, many women experience painful menstrual cramps. Even when the pain becomes severe, endometriosis may or may not be the problem. Perhaps because of this uncertainty, doctors hesitate to perform surgery to diagnose the problem until they have eliminated the possibility that the pain is caused by any of several other conditions.

A patient's complaint of pain during intercourse may be even more difficult for a doctor to diagnose. Not only is such pain hard to measure and evaluate but it may actually be caused by emotional as well as physical factors. This is not to say that the pain is 'all in the patient's head', but simply that its roots may be at least partly psychological. Even a doctor with experience in treating such patients may wonder if it is really as bad as she says, or if she is actually speaking, at least in part, from feelings of anxiety related to intercourse – perhaps because she has new sexual partners for the first time in years after divorcing her husband, or some other factor? How can the doctor know for sure the cause and severity of the symptoms, when all he or she has to work with are vague, subjective reports?

Infertility is another puzzling symptom. It is one of the most perplexing conditions facing the medical community today. A patient who tells her gynaecologist she can't get pregnant – she and her husband have been having regular unprotected intercourse for a year without success – may be merely unlucky. I have had patients who tried to conceive for three years or more without success. After attempts at artificial insemination and in vitro fertilization, they are ready to give up when suddenly the 'infertile' woman discovers that she is pregnant.

Infertility may also result from a low sperm count in the man or any number of other possible complications in the male or female reproductive system. Endometriosis is just one of literally dozens of possible causes.

As you can see, uncertainty surrounds a diagnosis of endometriosis by pelvic examination, ultrasound, and 'waiting to see' how the condition progresses. For this reason I feel there is only one sure way a woman who suspects she has endometriosis can know for certain, and that this method should be used to learn the truth as soon as the patient and her doctor have decided there is a reasonable chance that the condition may be the cause of her problem.

# Laparoscopy

The procedure known as laparoscopy determines not only whether or not a woman has endometriosis but how serious it is and how it may affect her fertility. Another piece of good news is that more and more doctors today recognize that laparoscopy is the only sure way of diagnosing endometriosis. This was not always so – and there are still many doctors who will try to diagnose the condition using only a manual pelvic examination.

By now many studies have shown that there is up to a 50 per cent error rate using diagnostic techniques other than laparoscopy, causing thousands of women to suffer years of pain and lose their fertility because their doctors did not take the trouble to find out they had endometriosis. For my part, I consider it an indispensible diagnostic procedure.

Laparoscopy is a safe, relatively painless test. However, it does involve the use of an anaesthetic (usually a general anaesthesic, meaning that you are unconscious during the operation), a small surgical incision in the patient's abdomen, and, in most cases, at least a day of bed rest followed by a week or two of curtailed physical activity. I have performed many of these procedures on an outpatient basis.

To prepare a woman who suspects she may have endometriosis, we have included a complete description of the laparoscopy procedure.

## The device

A laparoscope is a thin, inflexible fibre-optic tube about a foot long with a lens at one end that the doctor uses to look at the inside of the abdominal cavity. (See illustration on p 82.) The precursor to the device was an instrument called a proctoscope first used by Dr Bertram M. Burnheim at the Johns Hopkins School of Medicine in the USA in 1911. It was a thin rod that the doctor could use to look into the lower bowel through an incision in the lower abdomen using indirect outside lighting.

In 1912 a Swedish doctor by the name of Jacobaeus performed 115 examinations with the new device. A new lens system was added to the proctoscope in 1929 by a doctor named Kalk and in 1930 an American, Dr Ruddeck, recorded 2,500 procedures with it, using local anaesthesia and inflating the abdomen with room air for better viewing. However, the proctoscope wasn't accepted as a diagnostic tool for endometriosis until the 1940s, when Dr Albert Decker published a paper endorsing it.

From 1949 to 1967, doctors used an improved version of the device, called a culdescope. This was a quartz rod resembling a very thin telescope, developed by a Dr Gladu Forestier and his colleagues which offered much better resolution than the proctoscope. Light was transmitted along the rod from the near to the far end of the telescope, and photographs could be taken. This was the instrument with which I first actually saw endometriosis back in the 1960s.

The laparoscope used today is a refinement of this device and has been gaining popularity in this country since it was first introduced in the 1960s.

## The procedure

Laparoscopy is performed in hospital, usually on an outpatient basis. Most doctors schedule a patient for a laparoscopy first thing in the morning, and she is able to return home by the afternoon. She is instructed not to eat anything for a full twelve hours before the procedure and to drink only water after supper the night before.

The patient usually is given a general anaesthesic, and she is completely unconscious during the procedure. Some doctors, however, prefer to use simply an epidural anaesthesic, in which the patient feels no pain in the pelvic area but remains conscious. In that case, the doctor injects the anaesthetic into the space on top of the spinal cord lining. Having an epidural anaesthesia can be slightly painful, but some patients and doctors prefer to have the patient remain conscious during the procedure, which generally takes from twenty minutes to an hour to complete.

Once the anaesthetic has taken effect, the patient is placed on her back on an operating table with her legs elevated in stirrups, just as if she were about to have a gynaecological examination. Then the doctor inserts a manipulating cannula into her vagina up to the cervix. This instrument can gently move the uterus during the examination to facilitate visualization of the abdominal cavity.

The first step is for the doctor to make a tiny incision in the patient's navel. (The scar from this cut very rarely shows, even a few days after the procedure.) A needle is inserted and two to six litres of carbon dioxide gas are slowly pumped into the abdominal cavity. This separates the organs to allow for greater visibility. It may later cause some mild cramping.

The doctor then removes the needle and makes an incision half an inch long about one to two inches below the navel. This is to insert the laparoscope. One end of the instrument is sharpened, and the doctor gently eases this end through the incision and is able to view the abdominal cavity. Carbon dioxide continues to flow gently into the cavity through a sleeve around the laparoscope. Usually, the doctor will make another small incision a few inches lower down, through which a probe can be inserted to push organs out of the way for easier viewing. An assistant usually performs this task.

The doctor is now free to look through the laparoscope and all around the abdominal cavity. Endometriosis, if it is present, shows up as chocolate-coloured lumps, ranging from pinhead size to several inches across. Or, the growths may appear as a filmy covering over the organs and connecting ligaments. Either way, the condition is almost always easily recognizable by a trained doctor.

In a few cases, however, the adhesions are not dark but instead

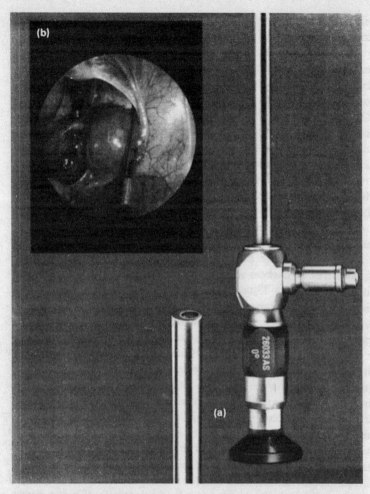

The modern laparoscope (a) is essential to the accurate diagnosis
of endometriosis. The laparoscope is inserted into the abdominal
cavity via a small incision. The doctor then looks through the
eyepiece and is able to see if endometrial implants are present.
(b) shows what the surgeon can see through the laparoscope. If
endometrial implants are present, the surgeon will remove them
using conventional or laser surgical techniques.

whitish in colour and diagnosis is more difficult, even with laparoscopy. Your doctor should be aware of this possibility.

It is nearly impossible to confuse endometriosis with an infection caused by pelvic inflammatory disease, or with lumps from cancer or fibrocystic disease, neither of which have the dark chocolate colour or clotted appearance of endometriosis. This is one of the main reasons laparoscopy is such a useful diagnostic tool.

Before finishing the procedure, the doctor will probably inject a harmless dye through the cannula into the uterus. The dye, usually methylene blue, will travel up to the fallopian tubes to determine whether or not they have become blocked.

It is very important that the doctor and patient have a talk before the laparoscopy to decide what should be done if endometriosis is found. In many cases it is a simple procedure for the doctor to remove the larger endometrial growths surgically right then and there, either by using a special tiny surgical instrument on the end of the laparoscope, by opening the abdominal cavity more fully to cut out large cysts, or with laser surgery. (See Chapter 8 for more details on this new procedure.)

If you are scheduled for a laparoscopy and your doctor has not discussed your options for surgical removal of adhesions, you should bring up the subject yourself. Otherwise a doctor may either not perform needed surgery or simply go ahead with a major operation while you are unconscious. Remember, the time to ask your doctor questions is well *before* you go under the knife. I am always amazed by the number of patients who tell me they never even discussed surgery with their doctor before they had implants removed. (See Chapter 2 for guidelines on communicating effectively with your doctor.)

A doctor should use this procedure as an opportunity to do a thorough search for any traces of endometriosis. Now is the time to find if implants are even beginning to grow *anywhere* in the abdominal cavity, not just in the obvious or clearly visible locations. The examination should look with equal care at both sides of the abdominal cavity, since the symptoms on one side don't always mirror those on the other (see Chapter 4). The *minimum* amount of time needed for a complete examination and recording of the diagnosis is about 20 minutes.

After the laparoscopic examination is completed, the doctor carefully removes the laparoscope from the incision, as well as the probe – if it has been used – inserted lower in the abdominal cavity. I usually suture both cuts, and generally all that is left is a small, nearly invisible scar.

In cases where there has not been extensive surgery, the patient is usually able to leave the hospital and return home within an hour or two of waking up. However, she should rest in bed for at least a day and will not be able to eat solid food for 24 hours. In cases where extensive surgery has been done I usually recommend that the patient spend one night in the hospital.

You may feel twinges of pain in the abdomen upon waking from surgery and during the next couple of days and some gas and cramping from the carbon dioxide. However, within five days you will be able to return to work and resume all normal activities, although strenuous exercise, such as jogging, swimming, calisthenics, or even brisk walking, usually are not recommended for at least two weeks.

Since a laparoscopy does involve surgery, it has certain risks. There are all the usual risks associated with being given anaesthesia – irregular heartbeat, overdose, etc. – but there is rarely a problem. There is the risk, although it is very small, of infection at the wound site and the instruments may perforate the bowel or bladder, resulting in serious risk of infection. As with any surgery, there may be internal bleeding during or after the operation.

You should keep in mind, however, that the possibility of any of these things happening is extremely remote, about one chance in several thousand. A doctor should make sure you know what the risks are – but also remind you that the procedure will enable you to discover, with very little doubt, whether or not you have endometriosis and, if so, how serious your condition is. You can have the results of the test immediately – in fact, your treatment may even begin while you are still being diagnosed and unconscious.

Most doctors will not discuss the results of a laparoscopy with you right after your surgery. If you have been given general anaesthesia the doctor will probably have left by the time you wake up, and even if you have had an epidural anaesthetic and remained conscious, you probably will not be in a position or mood to concentrate on a technical evaluation of your condition. Usually you and your doctor will speak on the phone later that day or the next morning. The doctor should explain how serious the condition is, and discuss with you any surgical treatment that was performed during the laparoscopy.

This is also the time to discuss all of your options for any further treatment. Some doctors and patients prefer not to combine laparoscopy with surgical treatment. If this has been the case for you, your doctor may then want to schedule surgery to remove implants, either by traditional cutting or with lasers. (Surgical treatments are discussed in Chapter 7, and laser surgery in chapter 8.) Most cases of endometriosis are treated with a combination of surgery and drugs, and both you and your doctor will probably want to start drug treatment as soon as possible after the surgery.

Usually the doctor (or, more precisely, an assistant) will take several pictures of the patient's endometriosis during the laparoscopy. I usually have the procedure filmed on videotape or have a number of pictures taken with a camera. If your doctor uses this procedure, as more and more doctors are, then you have a chance to get a look at the cause of all your pain and other troubles. Many patients find it reassuring to actually *see* what their endometriosis looks like – that it is not a complete mystery, not, as they may have been told, 'all in their head'. The condition has a name and an appearance. Ask in advance if a video or pictures will be taken, and, if your doctor does not offer to show you the pictures from your laparoscopy, you should feel free to ask to see them.

After treatment with surgery and/or drugs, you will almost certainly find that your symptoms will diminish drastically, and they may even disappear. However, the condition may return after as little as a month or two without drug treatment. Does this mean that you need another laparoscopy to diagnose your condition yet again? After all, the doctor should feel fairly certain that the same symptoms are caused by another case of endometriosis.

In general, if this happens I recommend that another laparoscopy be performed; however, whether your doctor performs another laparoscopy for a definitive diagnosis depends on the particulars of your cases. If you have had severe side effects from the drug treatment, your doctor may not want to put you on another course of treatment unless it's absolutely necessary. In general, a laparoscopy including cutting or laser treatment of larger implants may be performed instead. But a patient who has been better able to tolerate drugs or is reluctant to have more surgery may be put back on drug therapy within a few months without another diagnosis. As you can see, each case is different.

The important thing to keep in mind is that laparoscopy is the *only* completely reliable method of diagnosing endometriosis. Most doctors will not recommend the procedure lightly, since it is fairly time consuming.

The first time you report painful periods, pain during intercourse, or suspected infertility, your doctor will be wise to keep you under close observation for a few months before performing a laparoscopy. If pain is incapacitating (as in Jeanne's case in the prologue), however, or bleeding is profuse, a doctor should not wait but ought to act immediately by scheduling the procedure, especially if you have had previous treatments for the disease. And no doctor should prescribe any type of drug treatment for the condition without performing a laparoscopy.

Here we use two case histories to illustrate what can happen if the procedure is misused by a doctor – or not used at all.

Kathy was 25 when she first went to her gynaecologist complaining of pain during intercourse, but she said she'd been experiencing such pain for more than a year. The doctor suspected endometriosis and was so sure that without performing a laparoscopy, he gave Kathy a prescription for three months' worth of Danazol.

However, when Kathy returned for an office visit at the end of that time – 20 pounds heavier, depressed, and with an unsightly growth of facial hair – she reported that intercourse was still so painful that she and her husband had had sex only a few times since her first visit. Her doctor was puzzled but decided to keep Kathy on Danazol for another three months. He told her that perhaps her case was just 'stubborn' and slow to respond to treatment.

Kathy found that she could take only another three weeks on Danazol before she scheduled a visit to a different doctor, convinced that the first was not giving her the correct treatment.

The second doctor questioned Kathy more carefully about her symptoms and found that she had no pain at all during her periods. 'I haven't had cramps since I was a teenager,' she said. 'It's just during sex.' Tests for several pelvic infections and sexually transmitted diseases turned up nothing. Puzzled, the doctor suggested Kathy have a laparoscopy. Once the procedure was explained to her, Kathy readily agreed.

Surprisingly, the test revealed not a trace of endometriosis.

The doctor told Kathy that there was nothing physically wrong with her and suggested that she might want to seek counselling with a sex therapist. During her first session in therapy Kathy revealed that sex had been painful ever since a friend of her husband had raped her a year before – a secret she had been keeping ever since, unable to bring herself to tell her husband. Over the next few months, as she worked through the emotional trauma of the event and at last shared it with her husband, her pain gradually lessened. Several months later she reported to her gynaecologist that the pain of her suspected physical problem had disappeared.

Laparoscopic examination for endometriosis can also benefit patients for whom pain is a minor or non-existent symptom. At the age of 33, having been married for five years, Judith made an appointment to see her gynaecologist because for over a year she had been trying unsuccessfully to get pregnant. Her husband had already had his sperm count tested and had received a positive report.

After tests of Judith's hormone levels had shown that all was as it should be, her doctor asked her if she had pain during her period or intercourse. Not at all, she replied. Her doctor suggested that she wait three months and come back for further testing. She protested. 'I want to know *now* what's wrong.' Her doctor finally scheduled a laparoscopy.

The test revealed endometrial growths completely covering her right fallopian tube and ovary and two-thirds of the left. Fortunately, Judith's doctor was able to remove enough of the implants with laser surgery to feel confident that Judith could now become pregnant without having to resort to treatment with Danazol.

Happily, Judith found herself pregnant three months later, 'There's no way of knowing,' her doctor told me, 'but if we'd waited a few months before doing the test, we might not have been able to reverse the damage in time.'

As these examples show, laparoscopy is the *only* totally reliable way of diagnosing endometriosis. By actually seeing the disease, a doctor can tell not only how extensive it is but how it may affect a woman's fertility as well. A doctor can even begin treatment of the condition during diagnosis, using surgical techniques that are becoming more and more refined all the time.

While the procedure may bring slight discomfort and require the patient to curtail some of her activities for a few days, she will learn with nearly 100 per cent certainty whether endometriosis is the cause of her pain and infertility. If it is, she and her doctor have the information they need to take the next step: planning her treatment.

# Chapter 6

# MEDICAL TREATMENTS

A woman who has endometriosis – and anyone who is close to her – knows that diagnosing her condition is only the first step towards dealing with the problem.

Even though endometriosis has become a much more widely recognized and publicized condition, the search for ways to prevent, treat, and cure it has proved enormously difficult. And even now, many of the treatments still cause women almost as much anguish as the disease itself. Still, a great deal of progress has been made within the past few years, and prospects for future treatments look brighter still.

For most women with endometriosis, simply having their case diagnosed brings immense relief, emotionally as well as physically. After suffering for years from a condition with vague symptoms and no name, patients are relieved to gain at least some understanding of what the mysterious disorder is and to know that treatment will alleviate some of its painful symptoms. I've had dozens of patients remark, after I told them their diagnosis following laparoscopy, 'Well, now at least I know there's something wrong with me!'

The other side of the coin, however, is this: women find that the side effects of the drug treatments prescribed by their doctors continue to impair, in some cases seriously, the quality of their life. In addition, they know that while their drug treatment may lessen or eliminate their symptoms for a few months, it will not permanently cure their endometriosis. (The only true and permanent cure for the condition, as we have said, is menopause or hysterectomy.) Unfortunately, in the majority of cases, the condition does eventually return.

Various drugs developed to treat endometriosis do relieve a significant amount of pain and allow women who have been infertile because of the disease to have children. The price of treatment, however, can be severe depression, embarrassment, and even incapacitation stemming from side effects. The most common side effects, experienced by hundreds of thousands of women, are weight gain, fatigue, breakthrough bleeding, growth of facial hair, and deepening of the voice.

To help you find your way through the maze of drug treatment options, we have put together a list of the categories of drugs that are used to treat endometriosis, explaining how each one works, when and how it is most effective, and what its most common side effects are. Keep in mind as you read through this chapter that your individual response to a particular drug may be different from what is considered normal. It is important to learn the possible side effects of your treatment, but you should report to your doctor *any* effect you experience. For example, one woman wrote that after she started taking progesterone she noticed a change in her allergies. 'When I am on progesterone the allergies seem to be triggered by different things and I find I can be around or wear or eat things that I can't when I am not taking the hormone.' Although in this case the side effect was actually a positive one, it, like any other side effect, should be reported to the doctor.

The discussions that follow cover the generally accepted drug treatments for endometriosis, as well as a number that were used in the past and have now been discontinued.

# Painkillers

In the early 1920s, doctors' first efforts to treat women with endometriosis focused on trying to relieve their pain, the most obvious and debilitating symptom. (It was not at this time clear that the disease could cause infertility.) The standard treatments of the day, such as hot compresses and various herbal remedies, were commonly prescribed. These treatments, of course, did nothing to address the source of the pain but merely soothed it.

Several studies as far back as the 1960s have shown that analgesics, such as aspirin and acetaminophen, and the pain reliever ibuprofen can cause pain symptoms to diminish. Efforts were also begun in the early 1960s to treat the pain with the hormones oestrogen and testosterone (a male hormone found in small quantities in women), either in natural or synthetic forms.

In patients with stage one or stage two (minimal or mild) endometriosis, I have found that if hormone treatment is continued for several months to a year, the patient often is able to live comfortably with the condition.

Treatment with oestrogen or testosterone is especially effective when, during the laparoscopy, the doctor performs a dilatation of the cervix and removes some of the peritoneal fluid. This liquid is made by the lining of the peritoneal cavity – in which the uterus rests – as a result of blood being circulated through it. The peritoneal fluid contains 'scavenger' cells (see Chapter 9), lymphocyte cells, and cell proteins, all of which seem to proliferate in women with endometriosis.

Syphoning off peritoneal fluid during laparoscopy also improves the visualization of the uterus, ovaries and fallopian tubes. In general, I recommend the procedure, particularly in cases where the patient has been experiencing a 'lot of pain throughout her monthly cycle.

Several studies are in progress to determine whether the fluid of women with endometriosis is significantly different from that of other women, and if so, how. A 1984 study conducted by Shaki Badawi showed that the volume and types of proteins in peritoneal fluid change depending on the phase of a woman's menstrual cycle. The study also showed that removal of peritoneal fluid almost always brought the patient relief from pain.

Another helpful procedure performed during laparoscopy is the flushing of a dye, usually methylene blue, through the fallopian tubes to locate blockages and flush out loose bits of debris from adhesions. This procedure is not painful or dangerous and in some cases may help remove a build up of menstrual fluid from retrograde bleeding in the fallopian tubes. One recent study conducted by Malinak showed that these two procedures, combined with analgesic treatment, cause a complete or near disappearance of pain in 60 to 70 per cent of patients over a period of six months.

# Hormonal treatments

Patients with stage three or stage four (moderate or severe) endometriosis tend to fare less well with pain treatment drugs. However, medical science has attempted over the past 30 years to relieve at least partially their symptoms with a wide array of non-surgical treatments.

Since doctors discovered that the condition regressed when a woman was pregnant or reached menopause, and therefore was not ovulating, treatments have centred on attempts to suppress ovulation. This has been accomplished by administering oestrogens, androgens, progestins, or combinations of these and other hormones. Let's take a quick look at how these various treatments have fared.

## Oestrogens

Oestrogens cover a broad range of female hormones. The first efforts to suppress ovulation using oestrogens were made in the early 1950s. Doctors found that doses of one synthetic form of oestrogen, diethylstilbestrol (DES), at levels up to 100 mg a day stopped ovulation and thus freed endometriosis patients from their painful monthly symptoms. (The drug was also prescribed to thousands of women to reduce their risk of miscarriage.) The hormone also seemed to produce a softening of the entire genital tract, including the areas of endometriosis. Eventually, it was believed, the implants would be absorbed by the body.

Most patients, however, developed debilitating side effects from taking DES, including weight gain, bloating, nausea, breast soreness, vaginal discharge, depression, and irritability. In addition, it was later discovered that these woman and their future female children had higher rates of vaginal cancer if the women had taken the drug while pregnant.

## Androgens

These male hormones are produced naturally in the female body in minute amounts as a byproduct of the making of oestrogen. However, when prescribed to women in larger doses, androgens are also effective in suppressing ovulation.

Doctors began treating endometriosis patients with androgens in the 1950s. In a typical treatment, the patient would take 10 mg a day of a synthetic androgen known as methyl-testosterone for two menstrual cycles, skip a cycle, then repeat the dosage. Or, she might receive the hormone daily for 100 consecutive days.

Again, this treatment did what it was supposed to do in terms of treating endometriosis. Virtually all the women who were treated with androgens developed terribly severe masculinizing side effects – deepening of the voice, growth of facial hair, and severe acne (a masculinizing side effect even though women develop it as well; it is the result of a hormonal imbalance) – and most of them also gained weight due to water retention and the development of excess fat and muscle.

These side effects were so unacceptable and so universal that treatment with androgens stopped short of becoming doctors' standard prescription for endometriosis. I have not heard of a single case of them being used as treatment in the past twenty-five years.

# Progestogens

These are synthetic hormones developed to regulate fertility. They have been widely used in drugs ranging from birth-control pills to fertility injections. Doctors in the 1950s looked to progestins as a new, less debilitating treatment for endometriosis.

An attempt at a treatment that brought pain to manageable levels without introducing other unacceptable side effects was made in 1956 by a Harvard Medical School professor, Dr Robert Kistner. Observing that endometriosis patients who became pregnant had a regression of symptoms and, if eventually operated on, a less severe outcome with the disease, he had the idea of trying to introduce a 'false pregnancy' in patients for six to nine month intervals. The drug Kistner used was a combination of oestrogen and progestin that later became the prototype of the modern birth-control pill.

Kistner theorized that the hormones would not actually shrink existing endometrial implants, but that the tissue would no longer continue to be shed monthly. The implants would eventually outgrow their blood supply, die, and be absorbed by the body.

The theory worked in practice as Kistner had predicted. The most widely prescribed 'pseudopregnancy' drug was marketed as Enovid. It was administered in low doses starting at 2.5 mg a day for a week, building up over a period of six weeks to 20 mg a day, where treatment continued indefinitely, depending on the patient, for up to two years. This high dosage, by the way, has about 20 times the strength of the low-dose birth-control pills most women use today.

Another common progestogen used to treat endometriosis was Depo Provera, given in the form of injections every two weeks for four doses, then every four weeks indefinitely, with oestrogen added to control breakthrough bleeding.

Both of these hormone treatments caused nausea, depression, insomnia, vaginal discharge, and breakthrough bleeding, among other symptoms. On the other hand, they were very successful in treating endometriosis: more than 85 per cent of the patients experienced significant relief from pain. Even without the surgery that usually accompanied such drug treatment, many patients found complete freedom from pain for up to four-and-a-half years.

When treatment was stopped, most patients resumed their regular monthly ovulatory cycles, although some would not get their periods back for many months; a few for up to a year. Doctors did not anticipate this symptom and could not explain it. Many of them discontinued prescribing Depo Provera when they found unexplained and prolonged period cessation happening frequently among their patients. I still use Depo Provera to treat certain patients but never those who wish to become pregnant.

Doctors noticed that treatment with oral contraceptives generally did not work well for patients with large endometrial cysts. Even today, in fact, patients suspected of having such cysts should not be treated at all with birth-control pills containing progestin. I once heard of a case which helps to explain why I make this recommendation.

Carol, a childless woman in her late twenties, had been on oral contraceptives for five months. Although Carol had not been diagnosed with a laparoscopy, she and her doctor felt the treatment was 'working' because she'd experienced some lessening of her pain.

In the middle of one night, Carol was rushed to the hospital in severe pain. Doctors operated and found a large, two-and-a-half inch endometrioma ('chocolate cyst') had ruptured. The cyst, located on the abdominal wall, had not caused much pain until then. It had remained, however, because birth-control pills have no effect on such cysts.

The doctors surgically removed as much of the original cyst as they could, but the leaking fluid was not completely recovered. In subsequent months it formed scar tissue which worsened Carol's condition. She eventually needed another operation. Had her doctor been aware of the cyst and known that treating it with oral contraceptives was not effective, Carol might have been spared an emergency operation and months of additional pain.

# Pseudomenopausal drugs

High-dosage oral contraceptives as treatment for endometriosis came under attack in the early 1970s when research began to shed light on their dangerous – even potentially life-threatening – side effects. These included increased risk of heart attack, hypertension, and stroke. The findings received widespread publicity and set the stage for the introduction of a brand new drug treatment for endometriosis.

## Danazol

The new drug was a synthetic version of a male hormone, altered to reduce its masculinizing side effects, that was known as danocrine. Referred to as a 'pseudomenopausal' drug, danocrine (marketed as Danazol) works directly on the implants to shrink them, making it much more fast-acting than female hormone derivatives.

Danazol still carries with it many of the side effects of oestrogen-type drugs, chiefly bloating and weight gain. It also tends to cause hypoglycaemia, or altered blood sugar levels, which often results in lethargy and fatigue.

The following chart provides a comparison of the effectiveness and side effects of Danazol and oral contraceptive treatments.

Although Danazol is widely accepted as the 'treatment of choice' for millions of women with endometriosis, there are many women who cannot tolerate the drug and are unable to take it. As one woman wrote: 'Last year, I took danocrine (400 mg daily) for six months. My doctor said this was the last resort before surgery. The danocrine seemed to help for a while, but the side effects were so awful, I was miserable. Unfortunately, my doctor failed to tell me [about them]. I gained 35 pounds,

|  | Danazol | Oral contraceptives (Enovid) |
|---|---|---|
| Pain relief | 85%+ | 80% |
| Pregnancy rate | 50–60% | 20–40% |
| Side effects: | weight gain | weight gain |
|  | depression | depression |
|  | decreased breast size | decreased breast size |
|  | acne | acne |
|  | hair loss | hair loss |
|  | increased muscle mass | increased muscle mass |
|  | deepening of voice | hypertension |
|  | flushing | thrombophlebitis |
|  | sweating | increased stroke risk |
|  | change in appetite | increased heart attack risk |
|  | oily skin |  |
|  | uterine enlargement |  |
|  | swelling |  |
|  | fatigue |  |
|  | facial hair growth |  |

I was depressed most of the time and would often cry for no reason, and I started finding hair on my face and chest.'

As debilitating as these symptoms can be, many women are able to live with them for a few months to a year at a time. Some women are able to control symptoms of weight gain with a high-protein, low-fat diet and moderate exercise, although the validity of such efforts has not been proved by studies.

The best news about Danazol is that more than 85 per cent

of patients who try the treatment experience an improvement. Their pain symptoms are reduced or eliminated, and in many cases fertility is restored.

I have the results of a study conducted over a period of two years on 78 patients at all stages who were treated with Danazol. The overall success rate for pain relief was a high 82 per cent. Most of the remaining 18 per cent of patients had stage three or stage four cases. They may have experienced some pain relief, but the remission lasted only one to three months after the drug treatment was discontinued.

Doctors have found that the major advantage of Danazol over previous drug treatments is that by actually shrinking implants it can restore fertility to patients whose ovaries and fallopian tubes have become covered with endometrial cysts, which have prevented an egg from reaching the uterus. The pseudo-pregnancy drugs, on the other hand, merely prevent the adhesions from continuing to grow.

For example, one patient, 38-year-old Adrienne, had four courses of treatment with oral contraceptives. She had no children and she and her husband were extremely anxious to have at least one before Adrienne was too old to conceive and bear a child safely. However, after each treatment with the Pill, they were unable to achieve a pregnancy and Adrienne's pain returned within six months. Although she was reluctant to try Danazol because of what she had heard about the side effects, she finally agreed to try a six-month course.

The side effects were difficult, but not as bad as Adrienne had anticipated. The greatest benefit of treatment, however, was that within four months of finishing the treatment she discovered she was pregnant. She subsequently gave birth to a healthy baby boy, and a year later, a little girl as well.

Several studies show pregnancy rates of over 50 per cent in patients treated only with Danazol for minimal and mild (stage one and stage two) and moderate (stage three) cases. As a pain reliever, Danazol seems to bring significant relief in 80 to 85 per cent of patients at all stages.

Most patients take from 600 to 800 mg of Danazol a day for

six to nine months. The relief from pain is usually quick and dramatic, while the side effects build up over a period of three weeks to three months. For this reason most patients are initially very happy with the treatment.

The main problem with Danazol is the disturbing recurrence rate of endometriosis once treatment is stopped. About 20 to 30 per cent of women have a recurrence of symptoms within a year, and 5 to 10 per cent a year after that. However, if a woman is able to become pregnant in the intervening time, she will postpone the recurrence of symptoms even longer.

Patients with minimal to mild endometriosis (stage one or stage two) are generally put on a 600 mg regimen, while those with stage three (moderate) or stage four (severe) cases usually take 800 mg a day. Doctors have recently found that it is often extremely important for patients taking Danazol to follow their instructions for the proper dosage and timing of the medication to the letter, and that even small changes can make a significant difference in the effectiveness of treatment.

I discovered how important such timing was through the case of a patient several years ago. Lucinda, diagnosed with stage three (moderate) endometriosis, had been taking Danazol for three months and finding only slight relief from pain. She was on an 800 mg a day dosage, taking two 200 mg pills in the morning and two in the evening.

I did not want to increase Lucinda's dosage beyond the maximum dosage that I was prescribing to other patients. Instead I changed her schedule to taking one pill every six hours. Although this involved being awake at midnight and six in the morning to swallow a pill, for Lucinda the inconvenience was worth it: she immediately started to feel much greater relief from pain.

It should be emphasized – again – that Danazol *is not a cure* for endometriosis, and that as a treatment it is unacceptable for a significant percentage of women. If you experience side effects from the drug, you are in the majority, not the minority. 90 per cent of patients have significant weight gain (ten pounds or more), 50 per cent experience depression, and about as many get hot flushes. Many women are temporarily incapacitated by these side effects, just as they were by the symptoms of endometriosis.

Try to keep in mind, though, that for minimal to moderate cases (stage one to stage three), however, Danazol can be very helpful in managing endometriosis. Let us use a typical case, made from a composite of several patients, to illustrate the point.

Sally, a 22-year-old woman with a stage two (mild) case of endometriosis, took a nine-month course of Danazol and experienced no symptoms for four-and-a-half years. She finally had a recurrence a year after the birth of her first child and underwent treatment again. As her treatment ends she is deciding if she will try to have another child, which probably will postpone a recurrence of her symptoms.

Although it does reduce the size of endometrial growths, Danazol doesn't do anything to shrink masses of scar tissue formed by repeated deposits. Most doctors believe the drug is a vast improvement over the oestrogen-progestin pills it replaced because while the side effects can seriously compromise the quality of life, they are not life threatening. However, other drug treatments may soon be available that are even more effective – and less debilitating.

# GnRH

Doctors in the United States are now testing a new drug for endometriosis that has already shown promise elsewhere. Referred to as a gonadotrophin-releasing hormone (GnRH), it is a synthetic hormone that suppresses the function of the ovaries without the administration of oestrogen. In doing so, it is the equivalent of a medical oophorectomy, or surgical removal of the ovaries.

Studies using GnRH on patients with mild to severe endometriosis suggest that the drug shows promise. The hormone has none of the debilitating side effects of other drug treatments, such as Danazol. There is no weight gain, depression, or development of male sex characteristics.

However, there are a few other drawbacks. The treatment causes hot flushes in most patients, and it cannot be administered orally but instead must be given as an injection or a nasal spray. Also, several studies have shown disturbing long-term side effects such as loss of bone mass (which can contribute to osteoporosis) and thinning of the vaginal wall.

There haven't yet been enough studies on GnRH for it to be prescribed to the general population as a treatment for endometriosis. It does eliminate pain immediately and completely in many cases; however, its effects on fertility aren't yet clear. It also appears, like many other drug treatments currently available, to have a fairly high recurrence rate once the dosage is discontinued.

A review of the drug treatments for endometriosis seems to paint a somewhat bleak picture for the patient who hopes to reduce or eliminate symptoms through medication alone. A few patients, mostly those with only the mild or moderate stages of the condition, find that their symptoms do disappear for years after treatment with drugs alone, although their disease may continue or even progress asymptomatically during that time.

For most women, however, successful treatment means a combination of drugs and surgery, which is the subject of our next chapter.

# Chapter 7

# SURGICAL TREATMENTS

The goal of most surgical treatments for endometriosis is to remove as much of the disease as possible while still preserving a woman's ability to conceive and bear a child. As we have learned, this is not always possible. However, recent advances in surgical techniques to treat endometriosis – along with drug treatments – are allowing doctors more and more often to remove implants and adhesions while preserving fertility.

As a result, an ever-increasing number of patients are able to improve their condition to the point where they can achieve a pregnancy and carry a child to term. Surgery that preserves a woman's childbearing function is referred to as *conservative surgery*. It remains by far the most common type of operation for treatment for endometriosis. I believe that this should be the goal of the vast majority of efforts to treat the disorder.

## Conservative surgery

When is conservative surgery performed? Usually, when a laparoscopy reveals endometrial implants visible to the naked eye on and around the uterus, fallopian tubes, ovaries, and bowel. You should be aware that some doctors combine laparoscopy and conservative surgery. As a patient undergoing laparoscopy you should ask your doctor about this common practice when he or she schedules the procedure. (See Chapter 5 for a full description of laparoscopy.) This method is very beneficial because it can provide immediate relief from pain symptoms and, in some cases, restore fertility.

Whether surgery is performed during laparoscopy or in a separate operation, a skilled surgeon can surgically remove the larger endometriomas (chocolate cysts) in the abdomen without cutting or impairing the function of the ovaries, fallopian tubes, or uterus. Until quite recently, conservative surgical procedures were almost always accomplished with careful use of a scalpel, but now many doctors are finding they can operate more accurately, removing more endometrial tissue with less risk of infection, by using laser surgery. (See Chapter 8 for a complete look at laser surgical techniques.)

It is most difficult to preserve a woman's fertility when trying to remove endometriosis from the area of the ovaries and fallopian tubes. Doctors differ widely in their aggressiveness in surgically treating endometriosis in these areas. One patient wrote to me saying that after four years of infertility she was diagnosed with endometriosis and had surgery performed to free her left fallopian tube from the uterine wall. 'They were only able to loosen the end so it can sweep over the ovary,' she reported. As a result, the state of her fertility remained uncertain.

Conservative surgical treatments for endometriosis vary widely and are rapidly changing. Laser surgery, for example, was practically unheard of as a treatment for endometriosis ten years ago, and now thousands of operations are performed each year.

If your surgery ends up being performed at the same time as the laparoscopy, your doctor will not be able to tell you ahead of time the extent of the damage caused by the condition and therefore how much cutting or laser work will need to be done. When your doctor is viewing the abdominal cavity during the operation you, of course, are already under sedation. You and your doctor should, therefore, talk about possible options for surgery *before* the procedure is performed.

I often find, for unknown reasons, that patients don't seem to want to talk about surgery before they undergo it. Perhaps they feel it's bad luck, or they are simply too nervous for a rational discussion. I find, however, that once these patients do get talking about their imminent surgery they are full of questions. Many of them remark that they learned a lot and feel much calmer once they've talked. If your doctor doesn't initiate a discussion of your scheduled surgery, you should do so yourself. (See Chapter 2 for tips on how to talk to your doctor.) I usually have a pre-surgery conference with the patient to discuss the procedure, follow up, and possible complications, as well as alternative treatments.

As a doctor I find that I must not give patients any false expectations about the permanent relief they can expect from conservative surgery. In many cases, unfortunately, the surgical treatment of endometriosis turns out to be merely a stop-gap measure. It serves an important function, of course: repairing the visible damage the disease has caused and thus slowing its further progress. But often symptoms reappear at any time from a few weeks or months to several years later.

There are some patients, of course, who respond very well to conservative surgery. Their symptoms go into remission for years, even if they are put on only a short drug treatment programme, or none at all. However, I must stress that this surgery, like other treatments, offers no guarantee that endometriosis won't recur or even get worse. Each woman's response is highly individual, and you cannot expect your doctor to predict with complete accuracy the result of your surgical treatment.

The following chart, however, is useful as a general guideline. It shows the average rates of pain reduction and pregnancy following conservative surgery for the different stages of endometriosis:

|  | Pain reduction | Pregnancy rate |
|---|---|---|
| Mild | 70–80% | 60% |
| Moderate | 70–80% | 50% |
| Severe | fleeting | 30–40% |

A patient's relief from pain can last for years – or it may last only a few weeks. The average woman experiences six months to a year of relief, with treatment of milder forms of the disease resulting in longer periods than more severe (stage three and stage four) cases.

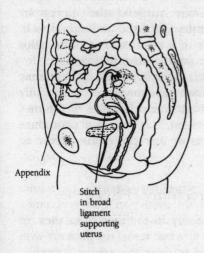

Appendix

Stitch
in broad
ligament
supporting
uterus

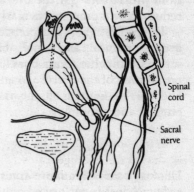

Spinal
cord

Sacral
nerve

*Figure 5* The effects of appendectomy and suspension of the uterus.

*Figure 6* Pre-sacral and utero-sacral neurectomy.

For most women, the possibility of even temporary relief from their symptoms and the hope of restoring or preserving their fertility makes conservative surgery combined with drug therapy the treatment of choice. A description of the types of conservative surgery that will most likely be available to you for treatment of endometriosis follows. I have at one time or another performed all of the procedures, although several of them, as noted, are no longer common practice.

## Suspension of the uterus

This operation is often performed along with surgical removal of the implants, and it is believed to help prevent recurrence of the disease and the formation of adhesions. In this procedure, the doctor takes a surgical stitch in the broad ligaments that suspend the uterus. This will tip the uterus forward so that adhesions are no longer able to form between the uterus and bowel.

Alternatively, the surgeon may suspend the uterus by stitching it in the back to the muscles of the abdominal wall. Both procedures put the uterus in a position that often helps reduce pelvic pain, particularly pain during intercourse.

The problem with both versions of the operation is that it may itself be painful, and some women have developed potentially serious difficulties with bowel obstruction because of the new positioning of the uterus. In addition, it is a surgical procedure and carries with it all the risks of any procedure involving cutting and anaesthesia.

## Pre-sacral neurectomy (PSN)

Doctors used PSN more commonly in the past than they do today. Now it is performed only as a last resort for patients with severe pain who do not respond to drug therapy or surgery.

The surgeon severs the nerves in the back of the uterus, which connect the sacrum (tailbone) to the internal os, which forms part of the ligaments that are actually part of the uterus. Cutting the nerves dulls pain in the pelvic area but since the suspending ligaments are left intact, the uterus is still held firmly in place.

Although a few doctors still perform presacral neurectomy routinely for patients experiencing even mild pain from endometriosis, it is considered by most doctors to be somewhat dangerous because of the risk of cutting blood vessels in the uterus, ureters, and colon. This, of course, can cause excessive bleeding, a very serious complication. In addition, the operation is usually effective for only three to four months, at which point the nerves regenerate and pain returns.

## Utero-sacral neurectomy (USN)

In USN the doctor cuts the nerves inside the uterus itself, making it a safer procedure now than it was in the past. It is performed routinely along with conservative surgery by some doctors. This procedure was first performed successfully in the 1950s, by Dr Thomas Doyle. It has been documented by Dr Doyle in *The American Journal of Obstetrics and Gynecology*.

This procedure, although it cuts the same nerves as does the pre-sacral neurectomy, cuts them closer to the uterus. Thus it affects more pain fibres in the nerve bundles. In addition, when the nerves are cut at this point, they don't seem to regenerate as quickly as the nerves in the ligaments that suspend the organ. As a result, some patients experience a year or more of relief from pain following the procedure.

There also appears to be less risk of accidentally cutting blood vessels than with pre-sacral neurectomy. The operation, when it is used, is almost always an adjunct of standard surgical removal of implants and drug therapy. You could say that it has been 'rediscovered' as very useful therapy.

## Appendectomy

This operation was performed quite commonly in the past, when doctors were more inclined to cut out the appendix for a variety of reasons, many of them unnecessary.

Today, appendectomy is performed primarily on patients with extensive visible endometriosis in the bowel area, especially if the appendix itself has been affected. The organ can sometimes be examined carefully during a laparoscopy. If so, the surgeon may judge that it is simpler to remove it than to excise implants, especially if it is covered with chocolate cysts or surrounded by a web of tissue. I usually try to save the appendix, and I find that the use of laser surgery makes it simpler and more routine to preserve this tiny organ.

## Microsurgery

Microsurgery has been used so far to treat only a very few cases of endometriosis. An intro-abdominal laser is used, one inserted laparoscopically, through an incision in the abdomen. It vaporizes implants at, but not below, the surface of healthy tissue. The type of laser used is designed specifically *not* to penetrate the tissue of the organs, which other than being covered with endometrial growths are perfectly healthy. The procedure maximizes visualization of small implants invisible to the naked eye. There is a very small amount of bleeding.

Although there have been no formal studies, evidence so far from doctors practising the procedure seems to show that there is slightly less risk of infection with microsurgery than with the still more common use of electrocautery (burning) for the removal of implants. However, the two procedures seem to be equally effective in preventing implants from recurring. Many doctors, myself among them, believe that, with refinement, microsurgery shows great promise for the future treatment of endometriosis, just as it has for treatment of other reproductive disorders.

With any surgical treatment for endometriosis, it is important to remember that the best chance of correcting the disease is with the first operation. Further operations may later prove necessary but are almost always less effective than the first. This is because scar tissue develops at the site of the burning of the surgical site as a part of the healing process, causing the organs to adhere to one another and making the future removal of chocolate cysts and adhesions more difficult.

One recent study followed 117 patients for three years and found that the recurrence rate ranged from 17 to 40 per cent after the first operation. However, it went up to 50 to 60 per cent after the second procedure. (The patients had been treated only with surgery, not with drugs.)

In almost all cases where conservative surgery is used to treat endometriosis, the operation is followed by a period of drug therapy that may last up to nine months. (For a complete description of the different drug therapies, see Chapter 6.) The two types of treatment, medical and surgical, are used together because they control different aspects of the cause of the condition, which is why you will probably need to have both of them as part of your treatment.

Drugs interfere with the production of hormones that doctors think cause endometrial implants to grow (see Chapter 3). Thus, they halt and sometimes even reverse the progress of the disease. However, none of the drugs currently used have a significant effect on large cysts (more than ten millimetres in diameter) which are usually made up mostly of scar tissue and only respond to changes in hormonal stimulation.

If not treated, these cysts can rupture, causing pain, infection, and spread of the disease. Even if they don't rupture, large cysts on the ovaries and fallopian tubes can lead to infertility if they block the release or passage of an egg.

Studies show that surgery alone, however, seldom brings a long-lasting halt to the condition. The usual result is a recurrence of symptoms, especially pain, for almost all patients within months (and many within weeks) of their operation. This is because the hormones are still acting to produce the same conditions that caused the endometriosis in the first place.

Since the implants that result from such a situation often cannot be seen, it is prudent to follow surgery with some form of drug therapy. When combined with drugs, relief can last for years and may, in a few lucky cases, be permanent. I treat the vast majority of my patients with a combination of drugs and surgery.

The biggest limitation of conservative surgical treatment of endometriosis is that it takes care of only what the doctor can see – the visible cysts and adhesions. For some patients, removal of these visible implants followed by drug treatment brings lasting relief of pain and restores fertility for a long enough period that they are able to become pregnant, even though smaller growths may remain. Other women, however, may have continuing symptoms even when microscopic endometrial tissue is removed. One recent study found that an electron microscope with magnifying power of 100,000 is required to see some implants under the lining of the peritoneal cavity in the back of the uterus. This area is the most common site of recurrence of the disease, partly because it's very difficult to see the area and excise implants there during an operation.

Fortunately, unlike infections, viruses, or cancer, endometriosis does not penetrate organs. Therefore, the damage can be removed from the surface by a skilled surgeon without harming the otherwise healthy organs.

Other, more radical types of surgical treatment for endometriosis are less common now than they were in the past, but are still used, particularly in severe cases. We outline these briefly below.

# Exterpetive surgery

Any type of operation that removes reproductive organs is referred to as exterpetive surgery. Hysterectomy is the most radical step, and the procedure most commonly performed to treat endometriosis is known as complete hysterectomy. This operation removes the uterus, ovaries, and fallopian tubes, and is used to treat advanced cases of endometriosis where pain makes it impossible for the patient to cope with day-to-day life. I consider hysterectomy a last resort treatment for the condition, to be performed in a very limited number of cases.

Most doctors today will try a combination of drugs and less radical surgery before recommending that a patient go ahead with a complete hysterectomy. The milder surgical and drug treatment will often reduce pain to a manageable level, at least temporarily. (See Chapter 10 for examples of patients who have chosen to manage endometriosis in this way.)

You should, however, note that *hysterectomy is the only cure – other than menopause – for endometriosis*. It eliminates the condition completely. This is because the disease is tied to a woman's monthly cycle and, therefore, cannot occur in women who don't ovulate and menstruate. (It's important to keep in mind that women who are amenorrhoeic, without a monthly period, due to low body fat or other reasons, continue to produce oestrogen. Therefore, these women can still develop endometriosis.)

If your doctor recommends that you have a hysterectomy as a treatment for endometriosis, you should realize that you must make a very serious decision that will greatly affect many aspects of your life, not only in the short term but for many years. Hysterectomy brings about instant menopause, no matter what your age. With the sudden onset of menopause you will experience hot flushes, vaginal dryness, and mood swings. This is because of the body's inability to produce oestrogen, the female hormone which controls reproduction, and also strengthens bones and seems to protect against heart disease. Having a hysterectomy also means that a woman can never conceive and bear children.

Hysterectomy cures about 95 per cent of cases of endometriosis. In the other 5 per cent of cases symptoms may recur, usually because a small piece of one ovary remains in the body cavity after the surgery. This may happen because the uterus, fallopian tubes, and ovaries are so covered with endometriomas and scarred by adhesions that it has become impossible for the surgeon to see them and remove the organs completely. Even a microscopic fraction of an ovary left clinging to the bowel or bladder will allow a woman to keep producing oestrogen – and allow the pain of endometriosis to continue every month.

I have heard of dozens of cases of this tragic result of

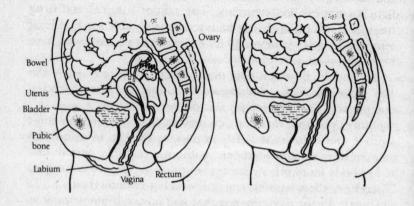

*Figure 7* (*a*) Before hysterectomy; (*b*) After hysterectomy.

hysterectomy. I know of one patient who had eight conservative surgeries and years of drug treatments for endometriosis to no avail. Finally, at the age of 32, her doctor performed a complete hysterectomy. The patient felt relief for the first time in years. Three months later, however, the pain was back. Although her doctor could not be certain, he told her that probably a piece of her ovary had been left behind after surgery.

It would be useless, the doctor said, to perform another operation, since the fraction would be too small to see and remove. The woman agreed that her only choice was to treat her symptoms with Danazol and ibuprofen to control the pain until she reached menopause.

Some doctors recommend that patients take oestrogen to reduce the effects of this premature menopause caused by complete hysterectomy. This practice is known as oestrogen replacement therapy (ORT) and many women continue on it for years after hysterectomy or menopause. However, you should keep in mind that the hormone may stimulate the growth of any implants that remain on other organs, so it is important to wait several months until all the implants die before starting this procedure.

It is also best to use a combination of oestrogen and progestin if you are on ORT, because of the association of unopposed oestrogen with increased risk of heart disease and reproductive cancers. The combination form of the hormone limits the activity of oestrogen for part of the cycle, giving the body a rest from the effects of oestrogen.

One 32-year-old patient of mine, after 13 years of oestrogen replacement therapy, developed a lesion in her vagina which became cancerous. This is a very unusual occurrence in a premenopausal woman. Such risks are actually quite rare, but because of even the slight risk of a problem associated with ORT, many women choose to try to get along without it after menopause or hysterectomy.

A recent article in the *New England Journal of Medicine* reported that oestrogen replacement therapy can help reduce the risk of osteoporosis (loss of bone mass) in postmenopausal women. Because of the new research, it appears that more women who have had a complete hysterectomy to treat endometriosis probably will be following the procedure with ORT. However, these women should still keep in mind that the therapy may cause flare-ups of their condition. Therefore, they might want to try simply exercising and, possibly, taking certain other medications as an alternative way of keeping the risk of osteoporosis at bay.

A complete hysterectomy is major surgery, requiring several days to a week in the hospital and up to a month of recuperation at home after that. The operation itself takes several hours and requires a great deal of patience and skill. There is a risk of injury to the uterus, bladder, and bowel, particularly if the disease is extensive and the organs have adhered to one another.

If you are faced with the possibility of hysterectomy, you should weigh the disadvantages and risks associated with the operation carefully against the relief from pain it almost certainly will bring. For the woman who has suffered years of debilitating pain, especially if she and her doctor feel that the disease already has made her unable to have children, the results of the operation may be worth the life changes it brings. This is particularly true for older women or those who don't want to have children.

If you are forced to make a decision about whether or not to undergo a complete hysterectomy, you should discuss your options thoroughly not only with your doctor but with friends and family, as the results of the procedure affect all aspects of your life. You should never hesitate to seek a second or even a third medical opinion. I always encourage my patients to seek a second opinion before they undergo surgery. Remember, it's your body and hysterectomy is your decision. Consider your choice carefully.

You will find, however, that more and more patients are now being treated with a new type of surgical procedure that allows for more precise, complete removal of endometrial implants with a much lower recurrence rate and less risk of scarring and adhesions. We move on to look at this new technique in our next chapter.

# Chapter 8

# THE NEW FRONTIER: LASER SURGERY

Laser surgery represents the latest development in surgical treatments available for endometriosis. The first procedures were carried out as recently as 1979 on a group of fewer than a dozen women with the condition, all of whom had previously tried other forms of treatment.

Actually, the first use of laser surgery for *any* medical procedure (in place of the traditional surgeon's scalpel) took place merely a dozen years ago. Since then, the field has shown phenomenal growth, and today lasers are being used successfully to operate on body parts ranging from the brain to the tiny bones in the hands and feet. Continued improvements of laser surgery techniques point to even broader applications in the future.

What exactly is this high-tech, futuristic-sounding procedure? Really, laser surgery is amazingly simple. The laser surgeon uses a very highly concentrated beam of light to 'vaporize' tissue cells. This simply means that the light breaks down the cell structure and suction is used to carry away whatever cellular debris is left. When treating endometriosis, of course, the laser beam is aimed at endometrial implants and adhesions.

Although there haven't been studies to show that laser surgery is any more effective than conservative surgery using a scalpel in reducing the long term pain and infertility associated with endometriosis, most doctors consider laser surgery the 'wave of the future' in the treatment of the condition. This is because they are convinced that laser surgical techniques will continue to improve, making them less expensive and easier to administer. Consequently, laser surgery will become more widely used as an effective and relatively simple treatment for endometriosis that can be repeated. Costs, as well as the risk of infection, should also continue to decline.

# Origins of laser surgery

How did laser surgery for endometriosis start? Laser surgery as a treatment for endometriosis was first described by a surgeon named Bruchat in France in 1979, when an attempt was made to vaporize large implants in about a dozen patients. The effort met with mixed success. The following year an Israeli doctor named Tadir successfully used laser surgery to vaporize smaller endometrial implants in several patients. The pioneers in the United States included Doctors Baggish, Daniel, and Pittaway. Although conservative surgery with a scalpel is still much more common, about a thousand procedures using laser surgery were performed in this country during 1986.

# How laser surgery works

In the most commonly performed laser surgical procedure, the patient is put under general anaesthesia, just as in a laparoscopy. Before using the laser, the doctor first makes a small, usually horizontal incision with a scalpel to open up the front of the abdomen – just as is done to prepare the patient for a laparoscopy.

Until recently, the entire laser instrument remained outside the patient's body during the procedure. It was generally positioned just above the abdomen. After making the surgical incision in the abdomen, the doctor directed the laser beam to any areas of endometrial tissue he could see. The drawback of this method, however, was that certain important areas remained inaccessible to the instrument, including the back of the uterus (cul-de-sac), which is a common site for endometriosis.

As a result, a new method that enhances visualization of such areas is now the standard procedure. The laser instrument is fitted with an inflexible fibre-optic arm – like the kind used in laparoscopy – that allows the doctor to actually insert it inside the abdominal cavity through the small incision. The two procedures are combined, and the result is known as laser laparoscopy.

I now make extensive use of this procedure in my practice and find that more and more doctors are starting to use it. It has generated a tremendous amount of excitement among doctors who perform surgery to treat endometriosis.

Laser laparoscopy has the enormous advantage of allowing the doctor to diagnose and treat the disease at the same time. The combined procedure saves time and money. Best of all, however, it usually brings the patient immediate relief from pain.

How does this procedure work? The fibre-optic tube sends a carbon dioxide ($CO_2$) laser beam from its top. (A more complete description of each of the various types of laser is provided below.) The tube is inserted into the small horizontal incision in the abdomen, and it can be moved by the doctor to various parts of the abdominal cavity. A doctor who is skilled in the use of laser laparoscopy can direct the fibre-optic arm anywhere within the pelvic area and vaporize endometrial implants without causing damage to any healthy organ tissue.

# The importance of laser laparoscopy

With laser surgery growing so quickly in use and the technique ever improving, I consider it paramount for a doctor who performs surgery for endometriosis to become familiar with the procedure and gain proficiency in its application. This is not to say that if your doctor is not using the procedure, he or she has a bad practice. There may be factors preventing the doctor from getting the equipment that are beyond his or her control. But you might want to suggest that he or she look into it.

Laser laparoscopy has many advantages over the earlier types of laser surgery – still in use among many doctors today – in which the entire laser instrument remains outside the body. First of all, it is smaller and more precise, and therefore can reach previously inaccessible areas. Second, because the surgeon makes a smaller incision, there is less risk of surgery resulting in infection. Third, laser laparoscopy allows the doctor to see affected areas, treat them and see the results immediately.

There is one disadvantage of laser laparoscopy that makes the procedure very difficult for doctors, and that is the problem of back strain as the surgeon bends over and peers into the laparoscope for long periods of time. A new method known as videolaseroscopy seeks to address this problem. Developed by Dr Camran Nezhat and colleagues at the Fertility and Endocrinology Centre in Atlanta, in the USA, this technique involves projecting a high-resolution video-recorded picture of the operation as seen through the laparoscope on to a screen. The doctor can look at this image while standing in a fully upright position instead of constantly peering through the instrument. In one study at the centre, doctors felt comfortable operating on patients for up to two-and-a-half hours.

# The effectiveness of laser surgery

Although no formal studies have been done comparing laser laparoscopy to the older, more invasive type of laser surgery, the technique so far has shown itself to be a safe, reliable, and effective method of treating endometriosis. I recently compiled the results of a study of 177 cases of patients treated with laser surgery over the past few years. Around 85 per cent had stage one, stage two, or stage three cases, and the remaining 15 per cent were stage four, the most severe. Every single one of the patients experienced at least *some* relief of pain following their first operation, and in most cases pain relief continued for a matter of months – longer if the woman was put on some sort of drug therapy.

For at least one of the patients in that group, the result of laser surgery has been more positive than she ever could have hoped. Eve Roth had had a laparotomy (an examination of the abdominal cavity, sometimes accompanied by the removal of endometriomas) before she became my patient. During the operation part of her ovary had been removed. She visited me because she was still experiencing pain and infertility. She was in her early thirties and she and her husband longed for a child. She had also taken a course of Danazol, which she said had relieved the pain only slightly.

I performed a laparoscopy with laser surgery. Eve's condition was stage three, with endometriomas covering both of her tubes and ovaries. I told her she had a slim chance of becoming pregnant, although her pain probably would be somewhat lessened because I had been able to vaporize many of the larger cysts.

Happily, Eve's progress confounded my predictions. She is now five months pregnant with her first child. Although most patients who undergo treatment with laser surgery are seeking relief from pain, the pregnancy rate following the procedure is high, about 40 per cent.

Doctors are now interested in whether or not laser laparoscopy will have greater long-term effectiveness than

119

surgery with a scalpel, and to what extent patients will have to follow the procedure with a course of drug therapy.

# The process of laser surgery

How exactly does the 'vaporization' process work? First any large or dense implants are excised and drained of fluid, which might otherwise leak into the abdominal cavity and cause inflammation and the development of adhesions. Then the laser beam is directed at one tiny area at a time, heating the small, concentrated area to about 2000 degrees Fahrenheit. The simplest way to describe the procedure is to say that the laser injects a 'burst' of energy into the cells, causing them to explode and release cellular debris. This leaves simply a cavity where the cell used to be.

The surgeon must use a tube called an irrigator to wash away the remaining cellular debris. Usually this is accomplished by making a small puncture in the abdominal wall through which the tube is then inserted. The irrigator, usually monitored by an assistant, creates a light suction in the abdominal cavity that sucks up debris as the surgeon works.

Use of the irrigator is important because any material that is left behind increases the patient's risk of developing further adhesions. The procedure also produces a small amount of smoke and gas (especially when using a $CO_2$ laser) which has to be periodically cleared away so it does not distend the abdomen or block the surgeon's view of the affected area. For this reason a laser surgical procedure generally takes longer to perform than surgery with a scalpel, which is usually completed in under an hour.

# What are the advantages of laser surgery?

The major advantages of laser surgery over standard surgical treatments are:

*There is less risk of infection*
A laser cuts and vaporizes endometrial cells without any instrument actually touching the surface of the tissue. This greatly reduces the risk of infection from surgery. It also vaporizes any other bacteria and many viruses that may have developed in the area. This is a very important benefit because the presence of endometriosis seems to make the pelvic area more prone to infection.

*The procedure gives the doctor more control*
Before the use of laser surgery, many surgeons cauterized endometrial implants away by using an electric current and many doctors still use this procedure. Cauterization is useful, especially in treating large cysts, but it has three major disadvantages.

- The instrument often sparks or jumps, presenting the danger of burning healthy tissue.
- Cautery burns below the tissue surface, deeper than the surgeon can carefully monitor, which can cause injury to healthy tissue.
- Cauterization can cause adhesions to form that are more readily at risk for infection and seem to heal more slowly than adhesions formed as a result of surgery performed with a scalpel.

The problem is that all of these possible risks are out of the control of the doctor and patient. Laser surgery, on the other hand, virtually eliminates all of them by giving the doctor much more control. The laser beam can be aimed precisely at the affected area, and the beam will not jump, spark, or vaporize tissue below the surface of the affected area. Each vaporization penetrates no deeper than one millimetre beneath the tissue surface, compared with up to five millimetres when cauterization is used. In most cases, no adhesions form as the operated-upon area heals, as often happens with conventional surgery.

In short, there are no surprises, either for the doctor or the patient.

### Laser surgery makes it easier to reach inaccessible areas

Doctors have found that the most important advantage of laser surgery is that it makes it much easier to get to implants in areas that are otherwise inaccessible, such as the back of the uterus, and to remove small implants from delicate organs like the ovaries, fallopian tubes, and appendix.

### Laser surgery is less costly

Though it comes as a surprise to some, laser surgery is, in general, less expensive than conservative surgery using a scalpel. Although the procedure may take longer (up to three hours is not unusual) because of the time needed to suction off cellular debris and wait for smoke and gas to clear, it is actually simpler than conventional surgery. It usually can be performed on an outpatient basis, and most patients need less anaesthesia than with scalpel surgery since the operation involves only one small incision.

It's important and interesting to note that the laser surgical procedure *itself* can be more expensive than conventional surgery with a scalpel. This difference in cost is one of the reasons scalpel surgery remains the standard surgical practice today. But as we have mentioned, most doctors who use laser surgery believe that it can be used on 90 to 95 per cent of their patients with all different levels of endometriosis. They also expect that refinement of laser surgical techniques will bring the price of laser procedures down over the course of the next few years.

### Laser surgery involves a shorter recovery period

Most patients need only a day or two of bed rest after laser surgery. The procedure is usually performed on an outpatient basis. If a hospital stay is required, it is rarely more than 24 hours. You would most likely be able to return to your job at least on a part time basis, within a few days after the procedure. With scalpel surgery, on the other hand, you might need to spend a few days in bed and not be able to return to your full range of normal physical activities for several weeks.

*Post surgical pregnancy rates may improve*
Several preliminary studies suggest that a woman's chance of becoming pregnant directly following laser surgery are much greater than after scalpel surgery. In one study, a group of women treated for severe endometriosis achieved a 55 per cent pregnancy rate within 12 months. A more recent study showed a pregnancy rate after 24 months of about 70 per cent in 102 patients with cases at all stages.

The recurrence rate following laser surgery appears to be about the same as that of scalpel surgery but doctors find when they reoperate, patients who had laser surgery performed have smaller and far fewer adhesions.

# Types of lasers

There are a number of different types of lasers in use today for treatment of endometriosis. They all accomplish basically the same thing and are used in the same way; the type of laser your doctor uses probably will depend on what is most readily available. Here is a brief explanation of the various types and their common usage.

*The carbon dioxide (CO$_2$) laser*
The most common type of laser surgery in use today involves a carbon dioxide laser beam. The instrument's only disadvantage is that carbon dioxide is absorbed by water, so the beam cannot be used to seal off large blood vessels since the procedure would involve a lot of bleeding. Since this often needs to be done when vaporizing large cysts, the carbon dioxide laser has been most effective in treating small cysts. It will probably remain the standard treatment for mild and moderate (up to stage three) cases of endometriosis because it is the most controllable type of laser.

## The argon laser

This laser is more effective in vaporizing large cysts. This gaseous laser cauterizes large areas of endometrial tissue and seals large blood vessels to minimize bleeding and the formation of adhesions.

## The NDG-yag laser

This type of laser is just starting to gain acceptance among doctors, and is still unknown to many doctors and patients. This type of laser has a greater depth than others and, therefore, has the potential to do a more thorough job of vaporizing an entire large implant. It can vaporize tissue below the level the doctor can actually see. However, there is more of a risk than with other lasers because the doctor gives up a measure of control of the depth of penetration of the laser beneath the tissue surface.

Laser surgery offers many exciting possibilities for the future treatment of endometriosis. Doctors emphasize, however, that the promise of laser surgery does not include a cure for the condition. Remember that besides complete hysterectomy (described in Chapter 7), no surgical treatment can cure the condition or guarantee that it will not recur in the future. But laser surgery shows the most promise of any treatment currently available for reducing your pain and restoring your fertility in the safest, least disruptive manner.

# Chapter 9

# OVERCOMING OBSTACLES: ENDOMETRIOSIS AND INFERTILITY

I am 28 years old and have been diagnosed as having endometriosis. I would like to have children but at this time it appears that I will be unable to. About six months ago I underwent a laparoscopy at which time I also had laser surgery to remove some scar tissue from my fallopian tubes. I just recently had a hysterogram that showed that my fallopian tubes are still blocked with scar tissue . . . I was told by my physician that further surgery could probably be done but there is only a 35 per cent chance that I will be able to conceive afterwards.

*A 28-year-old patient*

Doctors estimate that there are more than two-and-a-half million infertile couples in Britain. The term *infertile* has been defined to mean any couple that is not able to conceive a child after a year of having regular intercourse without using birth control.

It is thought that endometriosis affects up to 50 per cent of infertile women. However, if a couple is having trouble conceiving, it is not always easy to tell whether the cause of the problem is endometriosis (even if a laparoscopy is performed). This is because infertility is a complex condition in which many different factors may play a role.

Doctors who study endometriosis estimate that the condition is responsible for between 20 and 40 per cent of all cases of infertility. That means it accounts for at least half of all cases in which the problem is with the female partner. In fact, at any given time about 60 per cent of women with endometriosis are infertile.

The good news is that many of them, once treated, are eventually able to conceive. I have found that it's very important that you, as a patient, keep this in mind at all times. Many patients who have accepted the pain of their condition, the difficult side effects of drug treatment, and the trauma of surgery find the aspect of endometriosis that is hardest to deal with is that it has prevented them from conceiving and bearing a child. And for unknown reasons, women with endometriosis who do succeed in becoming pregnant have three times the risk of normal women of having a miscarriage. And this, of course, further reduces their chance of ever bearing a child. But by remembering that your infertility may well not be permanent, you will maintain a more positive attitude throughout your treatment.

First, however, you should learn how endometriosis can lead to infertility. Then we will discuss what doctors treating it can do to help improve patients' chances of some day being able to have children.

# What are the causes of infertility?

## Adhesions

In severe (stage three or stage four) cases of endometriosis (see Chapter 3), adhesions, or implants, form on a woman's fallopian tubes and ovaries. They can even exist inside the tubes. The adhesions, which are made up of scar tissue, often bind the tubes to the wall of the abdomen so they cannot move freely to receive an egg released by the ovary. If the adhesions form inside the tubes they can block the passage of an egg from the ovary

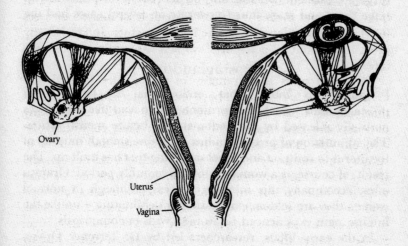

Ovary

Uterus

Vagina

*Figure 8* How adhesions cause
infertility by blocking the
fallopian tubes.

*Figure 9* Ectopic pregnancy.

down to the uterus. (This can also result in an ectopic
pregnancy, a potentially fatal condition.)

In some cases, the extent of the blockage is so severe that it
is impossible to reverse, even through delicate surgery to the
fallopian tubes. I have seen cases in which I will not even attempt
this operation because the damage to the tubes is just too
extensive. Although drugs and surgical treatment can remove
or shrink some of the adhesions, and thus reduce the patient's
level of pain, quite often she remains unable to conceive.

Surgery is usually more effective, however, in eliminating
infertility in patients with stage one or stage two (minimal or
mild) endometriosis than in those with more serious cases. In
studies conducted in 1984 by Dr Robert Kistner of the Harvard
Medical School in the USA, 76 per cent of 232 women with

stages one and two endometriosis became pregnant after surgical treatment, whereas only 38 per cent of 106 patients with stage three and stage four (moderate or severe) cases had the same outcome.

# Prostaglandins

It has been found that endometrial implants make prostaglandins, which are hormone amino acid-like substances normally released by the endometrium before menstruation. The stimulation of prostaglandins cause the smooth muscles of the uterus to contract and expel the lining that has built up. The result, of course, is a woman's normal monthly period. Cramps often accompany this monthly process, although in normal women they are seldom exruciating or debilitating – unlike the intense pain experienced by women with endometriosis.

In the early 1980s, researchers led by Dr Terrence Drake, head of reproductive biology at the American National Medical Centre in Washington, DC, theorized that women with endometriosis might have excess amounts of prostaglandins in their peritoneal fluid. These excess substances, they theorized, were stimulating the implants *outside* the uterus to behave in the same manner as the endometrium *inside* the uterus. Drake's study and several others since, proved this theory to be correct.

In one study, Drake and his colleagues collected peritoneal fluid from 66 women who were undergoing laparoscopy. They found significantly higher levels of prostaglandins in the peritoneal fluid of 32 of the women who had endometriosis, with the largest amounts in the patients having the most severe cases.

But what is the connection between prostaglandins and infertility? Although all the functions of prostaglandins are not fully understood, laboratory studies on animals have shown that they do influence various aspects of the female monthly cycle. In these studies, prostaglandins in the peritoneal cavity inhibit conception by causing the fallopian tubes to constrict and dilate very rapidly. These rapid contractions cause severe cramps and bring the egg down to the womb too quickly. The normal process of bringing a monthly egg to the uterus is usually timed so that, if the egg is fertilized, it comes into contact with the endometrium after it has built up and is ready to receive the egg. (If the egg is not fertilized, of course, it and the lining are expelled from the body.) It's interesting to note that this is why ibuprofen is effective in treating menstrual cramps in many women. The substance is known as a prostaglandin inhibitor.

If there is an excess amount of prostaglandins present in the reproductive system, the passage of the egg down the fallopian tube can occur too rapidly and the egg is too immature when it reaches the uterus to implant itself on the uterine wall. As a result, the egg usually aborts. Other studies have shown that prostaglandins may also inhibit the ability of the ovaries to release an egg, although why and how this happens is not completely understood.

As a result of these findings, the development of prosta-glandin inhibitors to treat infertility resulting from endometriosis has been an area of intense recent research. Some doctors have put their infertile endometriosis patients on a daily dose of ibuprofen, a mild prostaglandin inhibitor, to block the effects of excess amounts of the substances. However, no studies have confirmed that this is an effective treatment other than as a simple pain reliever.

## Luteal-phase defects

The luteal phase is the second half of the menstrual cycle, the 12 to 14 days after ovulation that culminate in menstruation. Because of the interference of prostaglandins and endometrial adhesions with the function of the ovaries and fallopian tubes, in some cases the development of endometriosis may start to throw off this part of the cycle. Either the luteal phase becomes too short, or inadequate progesterone is secreted to start the process that provides a proper environment for the fertilized egg to grow in.

As a result of one or another of these disturbances, the uterus is not able to build up a proper lining to receive a released egg.

129

Thus, even if a fertilized egg does get to the womb and implant itself at the right time, the endometrium has not developed into the proper environment to foster its growth. As a result, the egg aborts.

## Prolactin problems

Prolactin is a hormone that is secreted by the pituitary gland and helps to regulate ovulation. The substance has been shown by several studies to increase in women with endometriosis, although it is not yet understood why this occurs. One study, conducted in 1984 by Cecilia Schmidt and her colleagues at the University of Connecticut Health Centre, found that 20 per cent of patients with endometriosis had elevated levels of prolactin. This is a significant number. Clearly, the role this hormone may play in endometriosis-related infertility needs to be studied further.

## An excess of 'scavenger' cells

Endometriosis seems to cause an increase in the number of microphage cells circulating throughout the body. Known as 'scavenger' cells, these are a type of white blood cell, small in number but necessary to keep the blood free of debris. An over-supply of them, however, can throw other substances in the body out of balance. For example, they consume sperm – which can obviously have an effect on fertility. Scavenger cells also appear to be more mature in patients with endometriosis, which means they consume more. The name 'scavenger', by the way, is quite apt; these cells are voracious at any stage of their development.

In addition to consuming sperm, they bring about a decrease in the amount of hormones produced by the ovaries that regulate the luteal phase of the cycle. Doctors are trying to understand more about why and how microphage cells are produced in the hopes of being able to control their proliferation and effects in women with endometriosis.

## A higher rate of miscarriage

The miscarriage rate for the general population of women is under 20 per cent, but studies have shown that because of damage to the reproductive organs and disruptions to the ovulatory cycle, it increases to between 34 and 51 per cent (over half of all pregnancies!) among women with endometriosis. Obviously, doctors are concerned about this high rate and want to do what they can to bring it down.

Surprisingly, however, this miscarriage rate is highest among patients with mild or moderate – not severe – cases of endometriosis. Why is this? Because, as studies have shown, endometriosis causes luteal-phase defects in 62 to 67 per cent of patients, regardless of the stage of their condition, and these defects are the primary cause of miscarriage among all women. However, other factors often make it impossible for women with severe endometriosis to get pregnant at all. Since women with minimal or mild cases (stage one or stage two) are able to become pregnant more often than women with more severe cases, they also stand a greater chance of having a miscarriage.

# Diagnosing infertility

How do you know if you are infertile? If you visit your doctor because you believe that either you or your partner might be infertile, but you have not been diagnosed with endometriosis and do not know the possible cause of your condition, you will undergo infertility tests. The tests are not painful, but can be time consuming, and a few of the tests may be slightly uncomfortable. Therefore, it pays to know in advance what you should expect.

For the woman, infertility tests determine, first of all, whether or not she is ovulating. One test does this by measuring her progesterone levels at different stages of her cycle. The doctor takes two blood samples two weeks apart and measures the levels of the hormone. A significant difference between the two tests indicates that progesterone is stimulating the ovaries to release an egg, and that the egg is indeed being released and travelling from the ovary down the fallopian tube to the uterus as a result. Therefore, the cause of infertility does not likely rest with the woman's progesterone levels.

If you have endometriosis, however, this test may not tell you much about the possibility of infertility. The problem is that the absence or presence of a monthly cycle tells a doctor little about whether or not a woman's infertility is related to her condition. Studies have shown that up to 40 per cent of women with endometriosis do not ovulate, although many of them continue to have monthly bleeding.

Infertility tests also may include a postcoital check, in which a woman sees her doctor within three to four hours after having unprotected intercourse at the time of ovulation and has not washed or douched. The doctor takes a sample of cervical mucus, which is examined under a microscope to determine whether the partner's sperm have been able to penetrate the mucus and survive. If not, of course, the sperm cannot reach and fertilize an egg.

Another test, called a hysterosalpingogram, introduces a harmless dye, such as methylene blue, into the uterus and fallopian tubes and uses an X-ray to look for blockage of those organs. The test is performed within ten days of the end of menstruation. It is done as an outpatient procedure without general or local anaesthesia and can be somewhat painful. The doctor uses a small tube called a cannula to introduce the dye. It is iodine-based, so don't forget to tell your doctor if you are allergic to iodine.

None of these tests is particularly useful for diagnosing the endometriosis that may cause infertility. As we have mentioned, the condition accounts for 20 to 40 per cent of all infertility cases. More and more doctors are now realizing this, and as a result, many of them now routinely test for the condition – by performing a laparoscopy – in cases of infertility where a problem with the male has been ruled out.

I believe that a complete infertility check-up should include a laparoscopy, especially when other symptoms of endometriosis – such as pain – are present.

Here is a case involving a woman who became a patient of mine that illustrates the importance of using laparoscopy to test for endometriosis in patients who are infertile.

Sarah had been married and trying to get pregnant for three years, without success. She and her husband both had complete infertility check-ups, and both were pronounced normal. Yet Sarah still did not conceive. She had no pain either during or between her periods, but when her doctor finally, at Sarah's urging, performed a laparoscopy, the test revealed stage two (mild) endometriosis, which was completely blocking both her fallopian tubes.

Sarah was treated with laser surgery and six months of Danazol and became pregnant less than two months after completing her treatment. Routine testing for endometriosis allowed Sarah's doctor to not only diagnose her condition but also pinpoint the area of the problem and successfully treat it.

# Treatments for infertility in endometriosis patients

For years, doctors have told women diagnosed with endometriosis that they should consider having children as soon as possible if they want to have a family. After all, the chances of developing infertility become greater the further the disease progresses, and pregnancy puts the progress of the disease on hold, often making pain symptoms disappear until after the woman gives birth. But the woman who finds that she is already unable to conceive because of the damage of her endometriosis must try other treatments for the condition.

Surgery can remove adhesions (implants) from the fallopian tubes and ovaries, and in some cases the organs become unblocked and unbound enough to allow the passage of an egg, thus restoring fertility. In mild or moderate cases, a doctor carefully using microsurgical techniques (which are becoming more and more common) can create an adhesion-free milieu that allows conception to occur.

Despite the growing success of treatment through microsurgery, doctors are still recommending that a woman who has had surgery and wants to become pregnant start trying to conceive as soon as possible after the operation. There is a great deal of evidence that the adhesions start building up to their presurgery levels immediately after surgery, and I have seen cases in which they reach those levels within a few weeks.

Women who have been treated with drugs or surgery for mild to moderate cases of endometriosis find that when they do conceive, their chance of miscarriage is about the same as that of the general population. One patient of a colleague of mine, whom we'll call Jane, now suspects that she had endometriosis for years that didn't result in any pain but caused her to have two miscarriages. (She and her doctor never suspected the condition because not only did she report no pain but she was also able to get pregnant – twice.) When Jane tried to conceive the third time for a full year after the second miscarriage, she was unable to get pregnant and began having pelvic pain.

Jane visited her doctor, suspecting she might have endometriosis. A laparoscopy confirmed that she had a stage two case, and she was treated surgically and with Danazol for six months. She became pregnant five months later and delivered a healthy baby. Patients find that the infertility-causing effects of scavenger cells and luteal-phase defects are also eliminated once the condition is treated.

A word of warning: women who have endometriosis should be on guard against doctors and others who tell them that endometriosis is *caused* by their not having children. This is simply not true; women are predisposed to endometriosis for reasons that are not understood, but it seems clear that postponing childbearing can allow the condition to develop only in women whose genes already dictate that they will get it.

It is thought that the condition has become more common in recent years partly because its progress is halted during pregnancy. In times when women had larger families, and thus spent a greater number of their childbearing years bearing children, many were able to keep their cases of endometriosis at bay until they reached menopause, when, of course, symptoms gradually disappear by themselves.

Now, with the trend toward postponing childbirth and having smaller families, the woman who knows she is at greater than normal risk of endometriosis (because her mother, sister, or grandmother has or had it) or who already has it herself, may have to re-evaluate her plans for having children. Some doctors encourage such women to try to start a family as soon as possible, rather than waiting until the condition has developed to the point where they are permanently infertile. But it should be noted that pregnancy, like the more sophisticated treatments for endometriosis, does not 'cure' the condition but merely puts it on hold. It is for you, the patient, to decide if altering your plans of when you want to have children is an acceptable way to obtain temporary relief from endometriosis. It may be, but you should not feel forced into bringing a child into the world just for this reason.

As more attention is paid to the problem of infertility and more research goes toward probing its causes and searching for solutions, women with endometriosis can hope that they will have access to treatments that will prevent or reverse this most difficult aspect of their condition. From here, the prospects look good.

# Chapter 10

# A PART OF YOUR LIFE: MANAGING ENDOMETRIOSIS

I can only trust my doctor and hope that I will now enjoy my life . . .

*A 34-year-old patient*

The sentence above is part of the closing of a letter from a woman who had suffered, undiagnosed, with endometriosis for years. Like so many women, she had finally focused the issue of finding out what was wrong with her and getting it treated when she and her husband were unable to have a child. After she had eight endometrial implants removed from her pelvic cavity by laser surgery, her greatest wish was that she would be able to conceive before the condition returned. In other words, she was eager to get on with her life – adjusted to, but not defeated by, the fact that she had endometriosis.

By now it should be clear to you – if it wasn't already clear from your own experience – that endometriosis is a chronic condition. It usually does not go away. Many women who develop endometriosis are not 'cured' until they reach menopause or make the decision to undergo a complete hysterectomy, which brings 'instant' menopause at any age.

If you are lucky and seek out the best treatment, your endometriosis symptoms will probably be alleviated to the point where you can reasonably live with them, or they may even disappear completely. If your condition has not resulted in infertility, it is possible to keep symptoms in remission for a period of time by becoming pregnant (although this is *not* generally recommended as a treatment for the condition).

It seems that most women find that remaining in a state where pain is tolerable and the possibility of future fertility exists involves repeated surgery (usually combined with laparoscopy) and treatment with drugs. Women who are managing their condition in this way – and I have treated many of them over the years – effectively make the decision to live with endometriosis. They accept the condition as a part of their lives and make whatever adjustments are necessary – to their careers, family life, plans for the future, even where they live.

In this chapter we will share true stories of women who live with endometriosis. Their condition was diagnosed at various stages – from minimal to severe – and all continue to suffer to some degree. More importantly, however, they live with their condition, they *manage* it rather than letting it control or ruin their lives.

The feelings these women have experienced in their journey toward acceptance of their condition – and those they continue to feel, both positive and negative – are as important as the practical changes and adjustments they have made. The information is crucial for any woman who faces the possibility of having to live with endometriosis herself, or for anyone who knows someone who is living with the condition.

## Case study 1. Tanya W.

At 49, Tanya has had moderate endometriosis for over a decade. She was diagnosed with a laparotomy in her late thirties after several years of being unable to conceive. After three laparotomies she reconciled herself to the fact that she would never have a child. Her husband, however, could not accept the fact that Tanya was infertile, and so the couple eventually divorced.

Tanya was put on a six-month course of Danazol after each

operation. This kept her pain at bay; however, it would recur within six months, and she would live with it until she felt it was compromising her day-to-day life.

It has been almost a year since Tanya's last operation, six months after she completed her last course of Danazol, and she reports that she is pain-free. I suspect that this may be partly due to the fact that she is approaching menopause, as she says she is experiencing lighter periods. If so, she may never need another laparotomy or course of drug therapy. In any case, of course, there is no reason to operate on her as long as she is experiencing little or no pain. She asks if she is 'cured' – and I tell her she is managing her condition.

## Case study 2. Muriel S.

Muriel was diagnosed with moderate endometriosis four years ago, when she was 38. I performed a laser laparoscopy and prescribed a six-month course of Danazol. She was not able to tolerate the drug for even two months and did not want to take oral contraceptives since she hoped to conceive.

Muriel's pain returned and reached a level where she found it intolerable. This was a year after her first operation. We decided to perform another laser laparoscopy, which showed that the adhesions and implants had grown back into a moderate case of endometriosis. However, I was able to remove most of the disease.

The pattern repeated itself the following year. Muriel was frustrated that she had not conceived, but we both knew that she could not tolerate Danazol. (Her husband subsequently had an infertility check-up and was found to have a low sperm count. The couple have since adopted a child.)

This time, Muriel and I talked at length about the best ways to manage her endometriosis over the long term. She wanted to avoid a complete hysterectomy – which would bring premature menopause – if at all possible. She told me that she had not found laser surgery traumatic and could accept the prospect of yearly procedures to keep her condition under control.

We agreed to try this strategy. Two years later, we both feel that it is working well. Muriel accepts endometriosis as a part of her life – hardly the most pleasant part, of course, but something she has learned how to deal with. Although she keenly feels the loss of the children she knows she will never have, she finds that endometriosis otherwise does not exert a strong force in her life. *She* controls *it*, not the other way around.

## Case study 3. Stephanie R.

Ten years ago, at age 32, Stephanie visited her gynaecologist because she had been experiencing abdominal pain and was unable to get pregnant after two years of trying. The doctor suspected endometriosis and performed a laparotomy and diagnosed moderate endometriosis, with adhesions concentrated on the ovaries and fallopian tubes.

Laser surgery was performed three times before Stephanie was able to conceive and deliver a healthy baby girl. Two years later, after a laser laparoscopy, she became pregnant and had a second child just after her fortieth birthday. This time, however, her condition returned with incapacitating pain within three months of her delivery.

Since she had always been against taking Danazol because of its side effects, Stephanie decided that for her, the best course of action was a complete hysterectomy. A year later, aided by hormone replacement therapy, she feels she has adjusted to the effects of the operation. She is also pain-free and says she rarely thinks about her endometriosis.

## Case study 4. Alexandra J.

Alexandra is 23. Having experienced painful periods for years, she visited me, her gynaecologist, after developing symptoms of painful intercourse and pain during bowel movement. A laser laparoscopy diagnosed mild endometriosis and removed a number of small implants.

We decided to put Alexandra on a nine-month course of oral

contraceptives to prevent a recurrence of her painful symptoms. She was worried about Danazol's side effects and since she did not want to have children yet had no objection to taking birth-control pills.

About 18 months later, however, she did experience a recurrence. I urged her to try a six-month course of Danazol, which she tolerated relatively well. Now, six months later, she is pain-free. She worries that she will not be able to have a family. Although infertility is always a possibility, I urge Alexandra to try not to worry about it too much because I was able to remove so many adhesions before. In the meantime, she feels she is affected very little by her condition.

# Case study 5. Audrey S.

Audrey's case is about as severe as endometriosis can get. First diagnosed 12 years ago when she was 26, she had six laparotomies with no relief. A year ago I performed a hysterectomy with bilateral oophorectomy (removal of both ovaries). Still her pain continued to be severe.

Audrey is now responding to treatment with Depo Provera, given in the form of deep muscle injections. The shots themselves are unfortunately quite painful, but they bring Audrey relief from the pain of her endometriosis. We plan to have her continue with them indefinitely.

Audrey's case is one of the most extreme and debilitating I have ever seen and I want to stress that it is extremely unlikely that anyone with endometriosis will have to resort to the treatment extremes that she does – and still have to live with relatively severe symptoms of endometriosis. The majority of patients, like those described above, have periods during which they experienced virtually no – or very minor – symptoms, interspersed with times when their symptoms build to a point where they need further treatment.

The increasing ease of surgical treatment, the widespread availability of several forms of drug treatment that can be tolerated by most patients, and the spread of information available to women with endometriosis as well as the general public, are making these patterns of managing endometriosis more accepted and tolerated by women with the condition.

It is easier today than it was even two or three years ago for a woman with endometriosis to explain to her husband or boyfriend, her family, friends, and co-workers that she has this condition, that it is chronic, that it causes her pain at times, and that she may need courses of drug therapy or surgical treatments at various points in the future.

# Coping with endometriosis

By taking action to control endometriosis, you will most likely find that it is easier to live with the conditions it imposes on your life. This is not to say, of course, that managing endometriosis as a day-to-day, year-by-year part of your life is trouble-free. I can tell you – as you probably know already yourself – that there may be days when you will feel discouraged by the constraints endometriosis puts on you: the side effects of drug treatments, the curtailment of physical activities after surgery, the worries about your fertility. I think, however, that you will also come to find that managing endometriosis means a change in your outlook on your condition, a change to an understanding that you control it, not the other way around.

I have seen many women with endometriosis make this change in outlook. When a patient is first diagnosed with the condition, she is usually relieved to be able to give her symptoms a name, relieved that her condition is not life-threatening, and hopeful that with treatment she will become pain-free and protect or restore her fertility. She does not first consider the possibility of living with endometriosis, its symptoms coming and going at intervals, for a long period of time I find that it takes most patients at least a year, usually longer, to come to such an understanding of endometriosis.

I also find that when they do reach this understanding, it may have a direct and significant effect on their physical condition.

By realizing that you have a large measure of control over your pain and your fertility, you are likely to make much more of an effort to change your condition for the better. For example, if you are trying to decide whether or not to accept a promotion at work because you are worried that you may have a recurrence of endometriosis that was treated with laser laparoscopy followed by Danazol 18 months ago, you can weigh into your decision the knowledge that if debilitating pain does recur, you have the option of repeating the treatment.

It has been the examples of dozens of women with endometriosis I have known – and hundreds more I have worked with – that lead me to assure you that you *can manage endometriosis*.

# Chapter 11

# WHAT DOES THE FUTURE HOLD?

In this book we have tried to present the facts about endometriosis; unfortunately there is a lot more to say about what we do not know for sure than about what we know with certainty.

Such a state of affairs can be, as we have shown, a source of anguish and frustration to patients and their doctors. However, it also means that in the area of pure scientific research a lot of fascinating work has been going on concerning endometriosis (as it has been in many conditions related to infertility). We would like to leave you with some information and the latest updates on some of the most promising areas of investigation, which suggest what course prevention, diagnosis, treatment, and possibly even curing endometriosis might follow in the future.

## An endometriosis blood test

It becomes clear to anyone who is studying endometriosis – and of course to anyone who has it – that one of the reasons the condition is so difficult to diagnose, and therefore causes so much anguish to women before they even know the cause of their suffering, is there is no screening procedure that can be used to find women who are at risk.

A procedure similar to the simple skin test for tuberculosis or a blood test for AIDS or other conditions would tell women either that they were predisposed to getting endometriosis or that they already had it. It would also be useful in assessing the effectiveness of various treatments.

Researchers working under Suby Mathur, MD, at the University of South Carolina in the USA, have developed a test that shows whether individuals have severe (stage four) endometriosis. The test has been used experimentally to detect ovarian tumours by indicating the presence of a cancer antibody known as CA-125. In tests in the lab the antibody has proved effective in diagnosing about 78 per cent of ovarian cancer cases.

In two studies involving groups of 13 and 40 women, Mathur and her colleagues found that the CA-125 antibody test was also effective in detecting 80 per cent of cases of severe endometriosis and 49 per cent of cases overall. That means that the test has only a one in two chance of picking up endometriosis at any stage – not yet good enough to be used as a screening test for the general population of women.

It is hoped, of course, that as a result of this and other research, doctors will someday be able to perform a blood test on women to determine if they have endometriosis or are predisposed to it – just as your gynaecologist does a smear to tell whether there are cell changes in the area of your cervix that, unchecked, may develop into cancer.

# Tamoxifen

Tamoxifen is a new drug that has been used for several years in the treatment of metatastic breast cancer and has also been tested in the laboratory as a method of contraception. It is a non-steroidal anti-oestrogen substance that competes with oestrogen at various sites where oestrogen acts in the body, effectively blocking the secretion of the hormone.

The drug has been used experimentally in a small number of cases in which patients have responded not at all or with very limited success to other treatments. I have been using tamoxifen with varying degrees of success to treat four patients who are in the very rare situation of having developed endometriosis symptoms after hysterectomy (because a piece of their ovary remained, causing them to continue to ovulate).

Another study, already completed and published by G. M. Haber and Y. F. Behelak of Montreal General Hospital and St. Mary's Hospital, McGill University in Canada, reports on the successful use of tamoxifen to treat two severe, otherwise unresponsive cases of endometriosis.

The first patient, a woman, age 29, had a ruptured chocolate cyst on her right ovary as well as a smaller cyst on the left ovary and adhesions on the colon and cul-de-sac. After treatment with Danazol followed by surgery, a laparotomy found her still to have dense adhesions throughout the pelvic cavity. Her pain symptoms had worsened and she was unable to conceive. She was demanding to have a hysterectomy to relieve her extreme pain.

The other patient was a 24-year-old woman who, for six years, had been taking oral contraceptives intermittently to treat severe endometrial pain during menstruation and bleeding between periods. Laparoscopy revealed that she had adhesions throughout the pelvic cavity, especially on the tubes and ovaries, which were probably the cause of her infertility. She received an eight-month course of Danazol followed by a six-month course, to no avail.

Both women agreed to a six-month trial treatment with tamoxifen. Symptoms of pain and palpable scarring diminished markedly in both, and examination by laparoscopy showed only a few traces of 'inactive' endometriosis.

The women noted that the side effects of tamoxifen treatment were much less severe than those the women had experienced (and than most patients experience) with Danazol. Both women noticed hot flushes, particularly early in the treatment period, as well as fatigue and constipation. Neither, however, complained of breast tenderness, changes in their periods, deepening of the voice, hair loss, or acne, all of which are common side effects of treatment with Danazol.

With reports of only two women successfully treated with tamoxifen so far, clearly it will be a long time before the drug is offered to the general population of women with endometriosis. However, based on the success of the study summarized above and the anticipated favourable outcome of other tests involving more women, it is likely that larger studies will soon be run.

Therefore if you have, or know someone who has, severe endometriosis that has not responded to treatment with surgery or other drugs (such as Danazol), you may want to find out about the possibility of treatment with tamoxifen. Ask your doctor or contact the Endometriosis Society (address at back of book).

One problem that must be resolved before tamoxifen receives approval for widespread use as a treatment for endometriosis is the fact that since it does not suppress ovulation, women taking the drug could become pregnant. Experiments with rats have shown that the drug was given for a short time only (not more than a few months), and a number of the pregnancies ended in early abortions.

It is also not known what the long-term effects of tamoxifen are to a woman's reproductive system. There has been no demonstrated increase in malignancy as a result of usage in humans; however all reports have been in short-term situations.

Although more studies of Tamoxifen need to be done to determine its long-term effects and its effectiveness in treating endometriosis at all stages, the drug clearly shows promise for the future. With its smaller range of side effects and demonstrated effectiveness in treating stubborn cases of endometriosis in its most advanced stage, there is little doubt that doctors and patients will continue to look to the drug as a possible treatment for the disorder.

# Other possible treatments

What else might the future bring endometriosis patients, their families, and friends? There is hope in some quarters for a vaccine to prevent the condition, but no solid research yet supports the belief that such a hope may someday become a reality.

However, I feel this is a time of much progress for women with endometriosis. Advances in the precision of laser surgery make it simpler to manage the condition through operations. As a result, thousands of women have been given the opportunity to conceive and bear children – women who even a few years ago would have had to resign themselves to lifelong childlessness.

In addition, I see progress in the fact that endometriosis is becoming more widely known as a common condition among women in their childbearing years, a condition that is not deadly or dramatic, but that can severely restrict the quality of life. It is now more commonly understood that endometriosis affects not only the woman who has it, but also her friends, her family, her employer. This fact alone is tremendously helpful to you if you have endometriosis. It is simply much easier to live with a condition if those around you know what it is and how it affects you every day.

The progress made in recognizing, understanding, and treating endometriosis does not erase the fact that many unanswered questions remain. If you continue to suffer from endometriosis, the frustration of living with a condition with no known cause or cure never goes away. But the knowledge that millions of other women live with endometriosis, and that a great deal of progress has been made in facilitating your capacity for managing your case of endometriosis, all give you the power to make your life, with endometriosis or without it, as strong and positive as you want it to be.

# Glossary

*Abdominal cavity.* The body cavity between the rib cage and the pubic area that contains the reproductive organs, bladder, and bowel; the most common site for endometriosis.

*Acetaminophen.* An over-the-counter reliever commonly prescribed to treat pain symptoms in endometriosis. (Sold as Panadol.)

*Adhesion.* A mass of scarring, made up of old blood and produced by endometriosis.

*Amenorrhoea.* Cessation of the monthly period; occasionally an endometriosis symptom, but having many other more common causes.

*Anaesthesia.* A substance administered either orally or by injection to produce a complete absence of feeling during surgery or other normally painful procedures.

*Analgesic.* A pain reliever sold over the counter, such as aspirin.

*Androgen.* The male sex hormone; in the past synthetic androgen has been given to women as an endometriosis treatment.

*Appendectomy.* Surgical removal of the appendix through the abdomen.

*Argon laser.* A type of gas laser commonly used to surgically remove endometriosis.

*Auto-immune deficiency.* An inability of the body to prevent substances that are normally found in the body in controlled amounts from self destructing. One theory holds that endometriosis is caused by an auto-immune deficiency.

*Benign.* Not cancerous or malignant.

*Bladder.* The organ that collects urine before it is expelled from the body; it is a common site for endometriosis.

*Bowel.* The small and large intestine; another common site for endometriosis. In severe cases the condition can cause dangerous bowel blockage.

*Breakthrough bleeding.* A form of bleeding from the uterus between periods, associated with taking birth-control pills and with some reproductive disorders.

*Broad ligaments.* Bands of tissue that support the uterus in the back; a common but often unnoticed site for endometriosis.

*Cannula.* A hollow tube inserted into the vagina to facilitate examination of the uterus or injection of dye into the body for viewing other reproductive organs through X-ray.

*Carbon dioxide ($CO_2$) laser.* The most common type of laser used to treat endometriosis.

*Cauterization.* Burning with electric current or laser to remove endometrial adhesions or implants.

*Cervical mucus.* Secretions from glands in the cervix that vary at different times during the month and thus regulate fertility by blocking or admitting sperm.

*Cervix.* The neck of the uterus extending down into the vagina.

*'Chocolate' cyst.* An ovarian cyst filled with old blood and endometriosis.

*Classification system.* A system for identifying the severity of endometriosis.

*Conservative surgery.* A operation that prevents a woman's ability to conceive.

*Cul-de-sac.* The area in the back of the uterus and in front of the rectum which is a common site for endometriosis.

*Culdescope.* An instrument for examining the abdominal cavity for signs of endometriosis; it was a precursor of the laparoscope.

*Danazol.* The brand name for danocrine.

*Danocrine.* The generic name for a hormone-type drug commonly used to treat endometriosis by stimulating the conditions of menopause.

*'Deep'.* A term used to classify endometrial implants that are imbedded in tissue and therefore harder to excise.

*'Dense'.* A descriptive term for adhesions that are thick and unyielding.

*Depo Provera.* An injectable form of the hormone progesterone used to treat endometriosis in the 1960s, now not considered very effective.

*DES.* Stands for diethylstilbestrol, a form of synthetic oestrogen used to treat endometriosis and to reduce the risk of miscarriage. It was found to increase a woman's risk of endometrial, cervical, and vaginal cancer.

*Dilatation and curettage (D and C).* A procedure that takes fluid and endometrial tissue from the uterus to sample it; often performed as part of a laparoscopy.

*Electro-cauterization.* Excision of endometriosis with an electric current (rather than laser).

*Endometrioma.* See *'Chocolate' cyst.*

*Endometrium.* The lining of the cavity of the uterus; the material that makes up many endometrial implants. Adhesions closely resemble it.

*Enovid.* An early oral contraceptive also used in the 1950s and 1960s to treat endometriosis.

*Epidural anaesthesia.* A form of pain blocker administered by injection into the spinal cord and causing a cessation of pain only in the abdominal area.

*Excise.* To remove by cutting.

*Fibre optic.* A device made of glass fibres that conducts light, used to view the abdominal cavity in patients with endometriosis.

*Fallopian tube*. The organ (each woman has two) that carries a mature egg from the ovary to the uterus; a common site for endometriosis.

*Fertility*. The ability to conceive.

*Fibrocystic disease*. A very common condition in which lumps and benign cysts form in one or both breasts.

*'Filmy'*. A term used in the classification of endometriosis, referring to light, superficial adhesions.

*GnRH*. Gonadotropin-releasing hormone, a substance produced by the hypothalamus of the brain which tells the pituitary when to act.

*Hot flushes*. Temperature changes in the body that occur as a part of menopause; they are thought to be responses of the nervous system to a decline or absence of oestrogen.

*Hypoglycaemia*. Low blood sugar; a side effect of treatment with Danazol.

*Hysterectomy*. Removal of the uterus; called a complete or radical hysterectomy if the procedure includes removal of the ovaries which stops ovulation and thus is a cure for endometriosis.

*Hysterosalpingogram*. An X-ray procedure in which a harmless dye is injected into the fallopian tubes in order to view possible blockage by adhesions.

*Ibuprofen*. An anti-prostaglandin painkiller. Also available over the counter.

*Implants*. Islands of endometriosis, usually rather large, mature growths.

*Induction theory*. The theory that endometriosis is caused when cells change due to an infection introduced from the outside that repeatedly stimulates tissue surface.

*Infertility*. The inability to conceive after one year of regular unprotected intercourse.

*Infertility tests*. A series of tests performed on both the male and female partner to identify the cause of their infertility; more and more often the test includes a laparoscopy to diagnose endometriosis.

*Internal os*. The opening into the uterus from the cervix.

*Irrigator.* An instrument that washes the area of laser vaporization during laser surgery.

*Laparoscopy.* An operation that allows the doctor to see the abdominal cavity through a fibre-optic tube inserted through a small incision near the navel; the procedure is used to diagnose endometriosis.

*Laparotomy.* An operation used before the development of laparoscopy to see the abdominal cavity; it left a large scar.

*Laser laparoscopy.* The use of a laser (rather than a scalpel) to remove endometriosis during a laparoscopy.

*Laser surgery.* The use of a highly concentrated beam of light instead of a knife to cut tissue.

*Luteal phase.* The second half of the menstrual cycle after the release of a mature egg; lasts about 12 to 14 days.

*Lymphatic system.* A method of cleansing the body through the circulation of waste products, considered part of the body's defence against infection and disease; possibly affects the spread of endometriosis.

*Lymphocyte cells.* White blood cells whose function is to help preserve the body's immunities.

*Manual pelvic examination.* A routine gynaecological examination of the reproductive organs through probing of the abdomen and examination of the vagina and cervix.

*Menopause.* The end of a woman's fertility, occurring around 50 and brought on naturally by declining oestrogen levels or surgically by hysterectomy; defined to have taken place when there has been no period for a year.

*Metaplastic theory.* A theory that endometriosis is caused when the surface of internal organs changes because of chemical stimulus.

*Methylene blue.* A blue dye used in viewing the reproductive organs through X-ray for signs of endometriosis.

*Methyltestosterone.* A synthetic form of the male hormone androgen, used in the past to treat endometriosis.

*Microphage cells.* 'Scavenger' cells present as a cleansing agent

in the blood and existing in excess in women with
endometriosis.

*Microsurgery.* A surgical technique used on very small areas
with or without a microscope.

*Mild.* Stage two endometriosis, usually an early case.

*Minimal.* Stage one endometriosis, the earliest stage of the
condition.

*Miscarriage.* The loss of a pregnancy; more common in
women with endometriosis.

*Moderate.* Stage three endometriosis.

*NDG-yag laser.* A powerful gas laser recently introduced for
the surgical treatment of endometriosis.

*Oestrogen.* The female productive hormone.

*Oestrogen replacement therapy (ORT).* A drug treatment that
supplies oestrogen to the body in specified amounts when
the body is unable to produce it naturally.

*Oophorectomy.* The surgical removal of the ovaries resulting in
sterility and premature menopause.

*Ovary.* The female gonad, or egg-producing organ (women
normally have two).

*Ovulation.* The monthly process of making and releasing a
mature egg.

*Pelvic cavity.* The part of the abdominal cavity where the
reproductive organs are located.

*Pelvic examination.* See *Manual pelvic examination.*

*Pelvic inflammatory disease (PID).* An infection of the ovaries and
fallopian tubes, not necessarily serious but with the
potential to cause sterility.

*Peritoneal fluid.* Fluid made by the lining of the body cavity
(peritoneum) which in some women is affected by the
presence of endometriosis; a sample is often taken for
testing during a dilatation and curettage (D and C).

*Peritoneum.* The lining of the abdominal cavity.

*Post-coital test.* Part of the infertility check-up, it is a test of
the penetrability of cervical mucus at a woman's most
fertile period and is performed after intercourse.

*Premature menopause.* The result of hysterectomy.

*Presacral neurectomy*. The cutting of the nerves in the back of the uterus as a treatment for endometriosis.

*Proctoscope*. A hollow tube inserted into the rectum for viewing of the abdomen; a precursor of the modern laparoscope.

*Progestogen*. A synthetic form of the female hormone progesterone used in many drugs including the modern birth-control pills.

*Prolactin*. A hormone secreted by the pituitary gland to control milk production.

*Prostaglandins*. Substances found in smooth (involuntary) muscles which regulate their contraction.

*Prostaglandin inhibitors*. Drugs that stop the contraction of muscles; often used to treat menstrual cramps.

*Pseudomenopausal drugs*. Drugs such as danocrine (Danazol) that treat endometriosis by simulating the conditions of menopause.

*Pseudopregnancy drugs*. Drugs such as oral contraceptives that treat endometriosis by stimulating the conditions of pregnancy (cessation of periods).

*Retrograde bleeding*. Backing up of menstrual fluid into the fallopian tubes and out into the abdominal cavity; held to be at least partly responsible for causing endometriosis.

*Sacrum*. Tailbone.

*'Scavenger' cells*. See *Microphage cells*.

*Severe*. Stage four endometriosis, the most advanced and usually difficult to treat stage.

*Sperm count*. A measure of male fertility, performed as part of the infertility check-up.

*Stages I-IV*. See minimal, mild, moderate and severe; classification system.

*'Superficial'*. Endometrial growths just on the surface of organs.

*Suspension of the uterus*. An operation to reposition the uterus to relieve the pain of endometriosis.

*Tailbone*. The bone at the bottom of the spine.

*Testosterone*. A male hormone present in tiny amounts in females.

*Transplantation theory.* A theory developed by John Sampson in the 1920s attributing the cause of endometriosis to backing up of endometrial fluid into the abdominal cavity; see *retrograde bleeding.*

*Utero-sacral neurectomy.* Cutting of the ligaments in the back of the uterus (which can be done without major surgery during laparoscopy) to reposition the organ and relieve the pain of endometriosis.

*Uterus.* Womb.

*Vagina.* The female reproductive tract involved in intercourse.

*Vaporization.* The boiling away of the contents of cells through laser surgery to form steam and cellular debris; used to destroy endometrial implants.

# Useful Addresses

Endometriosis Society
65 Holmedene Avenue
London SE14 9LD
Telephone: 071-737 4764

Family Planning Information Service
27–35 Mortimer Street
London W1N 7RJ
Telephone: 071-636 7866

National Association for Premenstrual Syndrome
25 Market Street
Guildford
Surrey GU1 4LB
Telephone: 0483 572806

Women's Health and Reproductive Rights
Information Centre
52–4 Featherstone Street
London EC1
Telephone: 071-251 6332

# Index

157

# INDEX